WHY DO I KEEP
DOING THIS!!?

WHY DO I KEEP DOING THIS!!?

End Bad Habits, Negativity and
Stress with Self-Hypnosis and NLP

Judith E. Pearson, Ph.D.

Crown House Publishing Limited
www.crownhouse.co.uk
www.crownhousepublishing.com

First published by

Crown House Publishing Ltd
Crown Buildings, Bancyfelin, Carmarthen, Wales, SA33 5ND, UK
www.crownhouse.co.uk

and

Crown House Publishing Company LLC
6 Trowbridge Drive, Suite 5, Bethel, CT 06801-2858, USA
www.crownhousepublishing.com

British Library Cataloguing-in-Publication Data
A catalogue entry for this book is available from the British Library.

ISBN
978-184590732-7 (print)
978-184590789-1 (mobi)
978-184590790-7 (epub)

LCCN 2011938905

Printed and bound in the UK by
Gomer Press, Llandysul, Ceredigion

This book is dedicated to my mentor and cherished friend, Ron Klein, Director of the American Hypnosis Training Academy, who taught me hypnotherapy, neuro-linguistic programming, and much more.

Also by Judith E. Pearson, Ph.D.

The Weight, Hypnotherapy and You Weight Reduction Program: An NLP and Hypnotherapy Practitioner's Manual

Disclaimer

The contents of this book and the accompanying CD are intended for educational and informational purposes only. The contents should not be applied for the diagnosis or treatment of any illness or mental condition. No guarantees of results are implied, expressed, or intended as a result of reading or listening to these materials. The material is not intended as a cure or remedy for any disease, illness, ailment, or mental health problem, nor as a substitute or replacement for appropriate medical intervention. Readers who are under the care of a physician or other healthcare professional for any condition should consult with that provider before changing or modifying any treatment program.

The methods described in this book and accompanying CD are intended for use by adults and may not be suitable for children. The methods may also be inappropriate for people who experience hallucinations, delusions, psychotic episodes, or paranoia.

Author's note

Wherever I have mentioned experiences or conversations with clients in this book, I have changed the names and consequential details to protect privacy. Some cases are represented as composites rather than the experience of any one individual.

In deference to gender equality in language, I use the pronouns "he" and "she" interchangeably in this book when giving examples and instructions for specific strategies and processes. I ask that readers understand that I am in no way stereotyping one gender over another in my choice of pronoun. In applying instructions in the text to themselves, readers should simply substitute the pronoun of their choice.

About the CD that accompanies this book

The audio CD accompanying this book provides a guided introduction to the experience of hypnosis. The CD contains two tracks, approximately 4 minutes and 37 minutes long, respectively. Track 1 gives general guidelines for listening to the CD. Track 2 is a guided hypnosis session developed to help the listener acquire familiarity with the hypnosis process.

Track 2 teaches the induction/deepening methods found in Chapter 5: Eye Roll, Arm Drop, Counting, Eye Closure, Staircase, and Progressive Relaxation. In the Staircase induction, the listener imagines walking down a staircase onto a beach, and walking along the beach, seeing the sand, water, birds, and sky. Listeners with an aversion to staircases or to beach scenes are advised to forego listening to the CD. A brief, generic mental rehearsal follows the induction/deepening portion. The track concludes with suggestions for future success with self-hypnosis and a reorientation, with which the listener can return to full alertness.

Foreword

Last night I finished reading Judy Pearson's *Why Do I Keep Doing This!!?*, retired for the evening and slept very deeply. In my sleep I drifted and dreamed, and in the seemingly disconnected dream fragments a wise woman healer appeared amidst the saguaro cacti and blowing dust (I live in Tucson, Arizona after all!), and then the rain began, life-sustaining rain in the parched desert. Down from the mountains rushed the water, converging in the dry river beds, and throughout the land the shallow roots drank and drank. The healer gazed upon it all and smiled.

I have amnesia for the remainder of the dream but I can't help but remember the varied contents of Judy's book, which is nothing less than a remarkable achievement. If a person curious about hypnosis and self-improvement were to seek answers from only one source, it should be this book, which asks all the right questions and provides full and complete answers for one seeking solutions.

The companion CD nicely rounds out the total package and makes possible a post-hypnotic suggestion often uttered by the famous Dr. Milton Erickson, "My voice will go with you."

Now, learning self-hypnosis is not a magic bullet for, say, alcohol dependence or severe depression. With these and other common clinical disorders the author provides clear and careful explanations of other things the person should consider in addition to learning self-hypnosis. Judy, a seasoned practitioner who knows what she's talking about, makes it clear that some people may require additional psychotherapy and/or clinical hypnosis from a licensed mental health professional. I customarily tell my students, "If they show up and walk through the door, they're obviously interested, and the difficult part is out of the way." Kind reader, you have picked up this book and read up to this point, so you have taken that initial important step. You have entered the room.

The solution to your problem or my problem lies in the unconscious mind, and rest assured, Judy considered the unconscious mind in devising her techniques in this book. The solid writing and copy-editing make this a well-organized book that is easy to read and apply to your personal situation. Hypnotic content in a book allows you to discover and grow long after you've read it. It reminds me of the painter, Ted DeGrazia, who painted those pictures of the little Indians with no faces. When he put the final touches on a painting he said, "This painting is complete but it is never finished."

George Gafner, MSW, LCSW
Author, *Techniques of Hypnotic Induction*
Tucson, Arizona

Acknowledgments

I wish to acknowledge the staff at Crown House Publishing for their help in bringing this book to publication. First, many thanks to the Mark Tracten, the U.S. distributor who alerted me in 2009 that Crown House was open to a proposal for a new book on self-hypnosis. Mark works diligently for Crown House authors in the U.S., not only marketing our books, but serving as a sounding board and as our "ear to the ground" in the publishing world.

My heartfelt gratitude goes to David Bowman for accepting my book proposal. Through his expert advice and marketing savvy, I simplified and improved on my original concept. I am grateful to David and his associates for their forbearance and patience with my delays in submitting the drafts, due to the demands of my busy work schedule. Additionally, no author could ask for better guidance than that I received from Beverley Randell who gently guided me through the details of copy-edits and permissions.

It was my good fortune to work with Cory Foley-Marsello, the audio technician at Bias Studios in Springfield, Virginia who applied his talented expertise in recording and editing the audio CD that accompanies this book. He is a paragon of patience, who gave meticulous attention to every detail of the project.

My appreciation goes to George Gafner, an established author, psychologist, and hypnotherapist who graciously agreed, without hesitation, to write the foreword. I also extend thanks to Bob Bodenhamer, D. Min. for his straightforward advice concerning the length of the first draft. Both of these fine authors shared their own publishing experiences and gave me encouragement.

Lastly, I thank my husband, John, for his unflagging confidence in my writing abilities and for his continuing optimism throughout the production of this book. As an author with a full-time practice, my biggest problem was finding sufficient blocks of time to capture ideas on a computer screen and let my thoughts flow freely, without interruption or distraction. John, an author himself, understood this. He demonstrated unparalleled devotion by taking over several household duties, allowing more time for me to hunker down over the keyboard. Such a sweetheart of a guy!

I am grateful to the following authors who gave permission to quote from and/or adapt material from their publications:

L. Michael Hall, Ph.D. who gave permission to adapt the Neuro-Semantics Meta No/Meta Yes pattern and the Neuro-Semantics Mind-to-Muscle pattern from *Secrets of Personal Mastery*, Bancyfelin, Wales: Crown House Publishing Ltd., 2000; and the NLP Self-esteem Pattern from the *Accessing Personal Genius Training Manual,* Clifton, Colorado: Neuro-Semantics Publications, 2000.

Steve Andreas who gave permission to adapt The NLP Slender Eating Strategy and the NLP Responding to Criticism pattern from *Heart of the Mind*, Boulder, Colorado: Real People Press, 1989.

Carol Goldsmith who gave permission to quote from *The Book of Carols*, Haverford, Pennsylvania: Infinity Publishing, 2003.

Robert Dilts who gave permission to adapt *The Walking Belief Change Pattern* from an audio-recording by the same name, by Robert McDonald, Boulder, Colorado: NLP Comprehensive, 1979.

Nick Kemp who gave permission to adapt a submodalities pattern for negative inner dialog, from an electronic newsletter issued by Steve Andreas, 2008.

Jon Connelly, Ph.D. who granted permission to paraphrase a metaphor from his Rapid Trauma Resolution Training Program, conducted at the Institute for Rapid Resolution Therapy, in Tampa, Florida, 2006.

Rue Ann Hass who granted permission to adapt What is Your Soul Dream? from an article by the same name in *Anchor Point* magazine, Boulder, Colorado, 2003.

Ron Klein, who granted permission to paraphrase a quote from his Ericksonian Hypnosis and Brief, Outcome-Oriented Psychotherapy training courses at the American Hypnosis Training Academy.

Contents

INTRODUCTION

Are You Stuck In A Rut?

Do you keep doing a behavior that you dislike and want to stop? Do you have trouble getting motivated to do what you say you really want to do?

Do you, for example, want to stop smoking, yet you continue to smoke nevertheless – even when you know all the health-related dangers of smoking?

Or maybe you want to lose weight – which would entail that you stop eating the junk food and get yourself to the gym. Yet, in spite of the fact that you hate the way your belly resembles a kangaroo pouch, you nevertheless continue munching on the potato chips, slurping the sodas, and hanging out on the recliner.

Do you lose out on sleep because your mind-chatter begins in earnest when your head hits the pillow?

How about procrastination? Do you keep putting off that all-important project?

Do you worry needlessly, stewing in anxiety, when you could be relaxing and thinking productive thoughts?

And when it comes to performance challenges, like a job interview, public speaking, or sports, do you let your fears take over and ruin any chance of success?

Do you continually beat up on yourself and put yourself down, and then wish you didn't?

Do you ever wonder, "Why do I keep doing this?" If so, you aren't alone.

Even the saints, apparently, have wrestled with this all too common human dilemma. In the book of Romans, Paul wrote: "For that which I do, I allow not: for what I would, that I do not; but what I hate, that do I" (Romans 7:15, King James Bible).

I'm a licensed mental health counselor and life coach, specializing in hypnotherapy and neuro-linguistic programming (NLP). In over 20 years in practice, I've determined that most of my clients have one central problem: they say they want to *stop* a particular behavior and they want to *start* an alternative behavior, and they can't bring themselves to do either one!

Most of my clients are people just like you. They are smart, accomplished individuals. Yet they have a behavior, or an emotion, or both, that has run amuck. Most of my clients have tried everything imaginable to stop smoking, stop eating junk food, stop feeling nervous, stop procrastinating, and so forth – and yet they get stuck in persistent, unwanted habits. It drives people to frustration! So they come to me and ask, "Why do I keep doing this?"

Well, there is a logical explanation. What prevents people from doing what they sincerely want to do? What prompts people to repeatedly do things they sincerely don't want to do? To me, these two questions speak to a most perplexing facet of human nature that has bedeviled philosophers for centuries. Historically, scientists, psychologists, and physicians have offered all sorts of explanations, ranging from demon possession and childhood trauma, to irrational beliefs, personality types, genetics, and neurochemical imbalances. Some even attribute our neurotic compulsions to past lives or our astrological signs. To me, it all boils down to the fact that we aren't very skilled at managing our minds.

The Explanation Lies in Your Neurology

The reason why we keep doing things we don't want to do, or give in to inertia when we think about doing something new, can be found in our neurology. Even though most of us enter the world with a fully functioning nervous system, that system doesn't come with a user's manual. Even if it did, most people would never bother to read it. They'd stuff it away somewhere in the attic in that box of baby clothes and childhood toys.

The simple fact is this: neurology responds to repetition. Each time you repeat a particular behavior, or think a particular thought, or get into a particular emotion, your neurological system lays down a track in the brain's amazingly complex web of neurons. Do it often enough and your brain forms a network of connections around that behavior, thought, or emotion. It becomes "programmed" so to speak. Even your cells create new protein receptors to receive the chemical equivalents of frequent emotional states, and will demand more of the same – very similar to the craving addicts get for their drugs. Gradually, it becomes easier and easier to follow the dictates of our neurological networks and biochemistry.

When we try to break out of a habit, the "emotional" brain – the limbic system – notices that something is disrupting the status quo. It sends out signals of alarm and discomfort. We feel confused, awkward, afraid, or tired. The brain's language centers translate these signals into a form of self-talk that only reinforces the habit: "Oh, you don't have start that diet today! It's too inconvenient! Besides, it's too cold outside to go for a walk! Do it tomorrow! Here, relax! Have a cookie and stop thinking about it."

There is a solution, of course. This is to put the "logical" brain – your frontal lobe – in charge. The frontal lobe houses the brain's "executive function" with which we reason, set goals, persevere through difficulty, and achieve the outcomes we desire. To empower the frontal lobe requires that we recognize the limbic brain self-talk for what it really is – the discomfort of newness. Second, we must balance the emotional self-talk with a more assertive inner dialog based on affirmations, self-instruction, encouragement, and images of our goals. This is what I call "mind management."

Most of us don't think about *managing* our thought processes until it's too late – after addictions, habits, and emotions get out of control. Mind management isn't easy because it requires conscious effort. We find it much more convenient to avoid challenges, put off difficult tasks, indulge our appetites, give in to our fears, pop a pill, wallow in despair, and endlessly complain. Wouldn't it be nice if you could wave a magic wand and solve the problem? Well, we know that's not possible – but there is a way to manage your mind effectively with self-hypnosis.

Why Self-Hypnosis?

I once had a booth at a local health fair where I displayed brochures about my practice and pamphlets about my upcoming self-hypnosis class. A nicely-dressed man walked by my table and said to his companion, "Hypnosis! No one can tell *me* how to think! I don't want anyone messing with my mind!"

I said nothing and the man walked away. I felt sorry for him, in a way, because first of all, hypnosis is not "messing with the mind." It's a proven way for teaching people how to manage their thinking so that they achieve more of what they want out of life. It's an established method for instilling confidence, releasing unwanted habits, managing pain, and promoting relaxation. It improves coping mechanisms, speeds healing from injury, and helps people acquire self-discipline. Hypnosis capitalizes on the magic of imagination, relying on self-talk and internal imagery, thereby facilitating mind-body communication. While most people think hypnosis takes away self-control, the opposite is true. Hypnosis restores self-control! That man didn't know what he was missing out on!

Hypnosis is the best way I know to teach people how to manage their thinking and direct the mind productively. Hypnosis relaxes and quiets the chatter of the mind, so that we can speak to ourselves logically and concentrate on solutions. Hypnosis has a specific positive effect on the brain and gives it a clear channel for communicating with the body. Hypnosis is an excellent vehicle for visualization – visualizing goals, new behaviors, and healing processes. Hypnosis allows people to interrupt the patterns that keep them stuck. Hypnosis provides strategies to manage the mind to access the qualities and strengths you already possess.

NLP is the psychological approach that spells out those strategies step-by-step. NLP combines trance-work with specific cognitive processes that help people to access resourceful states, mentally practice those states, and apply those states, later, in real-life circumstances. In this book, I'll explain how the concepts and mechanisms of hypnosis and the principles of NLP make for effective approaches to self-hypnosis.

Self-hypnosis costs nothing except the time it takes to do it. The tools of self-hypnosis are as close at hand as the next quiet moment. With self-hypnosis, you can learn how to manage your mind to stop doing what you don't like and start doing what you say you want to do. With the focus that self-hypnosis provides, you can engage in the visualizations, the affirmations, and the mental practice that lays down new neurological connections and pathways.

The Better Question

It might surprise you to discover that when it comes to changing unwanted behaviors and emotions and adapting new ones, "Why do I keep doing this?" isn't the best question. Knowing why doesn't always lead to a solution. Having an explanation may help, but it doesn't teach you what to *do* to solve the problem. Asking "Why?" will keep you focused on the problem, not the solution.

There is a better question that targets the solution, which is "How can I solve this?" That's what this book is all about – solutions based on step-by-step self-hypnosis strategies. This book will give you the tools and processes for managing your mind so that you free yourself from unwanted habits, accomplish the outcomes you want, and utilize more of your talents and potentials.

In Part I of this book, you'll find basic information about hypnosis and NLP. You'll learn easy methods for going into trance, visualizing results, giving yourself suggestions, and coming out of trance. The CD that accompanies this book features a self-hypnosis training trance that guides you through various methods of trance induction and deepening.

For Part II, I've chosen the 16 self-hypnosis applications that individuals most often bring to hypnotherapy. These are the typical problems and concerns that I've helped my clients solve for over two decades. With each application, I've included practical behavioral advice as well as step-by-step self-hypnosis strategies. The applications cover problematic issues such as habits and addictions, smoking, overeating, insomnia, procrastination, emotional difficulties, and pain management, as well as personal growth outcomes such as improved performance, better self-esteem, accessing your intuition, and discovering your life purpose.

I hope that when you read this book, you'll bring to it a specific goal. Please look upon this book as an opportunity to come to terms with an unwanted habit, negative thinking, irrational fears, or some other form of self-sabotage. I also hope you'll find in this book a number of simple guidelines for transforming the quality of your life. With the skills and information herein, you can learn to maintain equanimity in the face of challenges, direct your thinking more effectively, and develop resilience in response to adversity. I would feel gratified beyond measure if this book becomes one that you turn to, from time to time, as a trusted source of guidance for future issues as they arise.

PART I

What You Need
to Know Before You Start
Self-Hypnosis

If you decided to read this book to solve a specific problem, you'd probably like to jump ahead to Part II to get started on self-hypnosis right away. However, I invite you to read Part I first, for a fuller understanding about hypnosis than you might currently possess. I also suggest that you read these first five chapters before listening to the CD that accompanies the book. With this preliminary information, I believe you will approach self-hypnosis more confidently and competently than otherwise.

Of course, if you are trained in hypnosis, the initial five chapters will be "old hat" to you. You will probably want to skip them. However, if you are a novice to hypnosis, then Part I will simplify and demystify the hypnotic process for you.

Chapter 1 begins with a brief history of hypnosis, highlighting the work of two of the most influential hypnotherapists of the twentieth century: Milton H. Erickson and Dave Elman. Each had a unique approach to hypnosis. Their influence continues today, long after their deaths. Chapter 2 explores what hypnosis is, with information on trance, hypnosis and the brain, and hypnotizability. I will reveal to you how to avoid the one problem that will most likely defeat your attempts at self-hypnosis.

When I started training in clinical hypnosis over 20 years ago, I learned it through NLP practitioner training. Frankly, I can't imagine doing hypnosis without knowing NLP, so that's the topic of Chapter 3. NLP distills cognitive-behavioral change into a series of mental steps that produce reliable, time-tested strategies. Without such strategies, hypnosis gives people suggestions about what to do without telling them specifically *how* to organize their thinking in order to do it. With NLP, you'll learn self-hypnosis strategies that bring real results!

Chapter 4 is about the nuts and bolts of hypnosis: affirmations and visualization. We think and communicate to ourselves and others through words and pictures. Affirmations are suggestions you'll give yourself in trance. Visualization constitutes the pictures and movies you'll make in your mind during self-hypnosis. With words and pictures, your mind reshapes physical responses in the brain and the body.

Chapter 5 is about inducing and deepening trance. This chapter explains the entire self-hypnosis process from beginning to end: how to get into trance, what to do in trance, and how to get out of trance. I'll give you ideas for recording your own self-hypnosis sessions. I'll also tell you how to locate a good hypnotherapist, in case you want to work with a professional.

In these first five chapters I've done my best to give solid, useful information, without getting too technical or overly academic. I've also made every effort to avoid the tawdry marketing hype and false claims made by so many self-proclaimed gurus of hypnosis. My intention is to teach you everything *you* should know, without teaching you everything *I* know. Nevertheless, I hope to convey to you my own fascination with NLP, hypnosis, and the mind. I hope you'll come to share that fascination with me.

CHAPTER 1

Hypnosis: Where Did it Come From?

For centuries, various cultures have used trance and altered states of consciousness in ceremonial rituals and healing. The ancient Greeks, for example, erected healing temples where the weary and the sick could go to rest: where Hypnos, the god of sleep, removed their cares and pain. Egyptians and Hindus had similar customs.

Modern-day hypnosis began in France, with a German-born physician; Franz Anton Mesmer (1734–1815). He developed a therapeutic method in which he passed his hands over the body of a patient, at which point the patient swooned into trance. He believed his method balanced body energies – something he called "animal magnetism." "Mesmerism," as his work came to be called, brought about several cures. However, in 1784, the monarchy called for a commission to investigate Mesmer's claims. After a number of inquiries, the commission concluded that there was no evidence for animal magnetism. Mesmer's cures were attributed to "imagination" – what today, we might call "the placebo effect." Mesmer soon retired and little is known about the remaining years of his life.

A few physicians throughout Europe continued to use Mesmer's methods, finding that their patients would usually swoon into a sleep-like state and emerge feeling better. These physicians found that they could use trance-inducing methods to perform painless surgeries without anesthesia. In 1841, Scottish surgeon James Braid (1795–1860), upon witnessing a demonstration of mesmerism, renamed the process "hypnotism." He was convinced that hypnotic trance was due to a natural psychological process involving concentration and visualization. He was right.

The First International Congress for Experimental and Therapeutic Hypnotism was held in Paris in 1889. In 1892, the British Medical Association endorsed hypnosis for therapeutic applications. Although hypnosis had promising beginnings, medical schools and universities largely ignored the subject.

Hypnosis lacked academic respectability mainly because of the way in which hypnotic methods had evolved. Traditional hypnosis consisted of a direct, authoritarian, repetitive approach. Patients were commanded to "sleep." Few people could be hypnotized in this manner. With hypnosis seeming so unreliable, many physicians regarded it as useless. Others suspected that hypnotic subjects were faking trance or acting out of social compliance, or that hypnosis worked only on "imagined" illnesses.

However, in 1933, an American psychologist, Clark Hull (1884–1952), published *Hypnosis and Suggestibility*, a rigorous study of hypnosis, reporting on statistical and experimental analyses.[1] Hull's studies demonstrated that the hypnotic state was not sleep. He documented several effects of hypnosis, such as pain control, stating that suggestion and the subject's motivation were major factors in the success of hypnosis.

From the 1930s onward, hypnosis became a topic of psychological research, particularly in the U.S., the U.K., and Europe. Researchers developed tests to measure suggestibility and hypnotizability. Hypnosis gradually found its way into the practice of general psychiatry, mostly for patients in inpatient settings and mental institutions.

Erickson and Elman

In the mid-twentieth century, two major figures revolutionized the practice of clinical hypnosis, propelling it into prominence as a recognized specialty in medicine and psychology. These influences came from Milton H. Erickson, M.D. (1901–1980) and Dave Elman (1900–1967).

Erickson was an innovative clinician. He was known for his "utilization" approach, in which he adapted his instructions, recommendations, and assignments to the personality, interests, and characteristics of each patient. He "utilized" whatever each patient presented, or whatever made each patient unique, as a vehicle for suggesting and influencing change. He gave his patients interesting and unusual assignments, implying that the tasks held valuable lessons. He advised patients to make small changes that often led to much more significant transformation.

Unlike traditional hypnotherapists, Erickson conducted hypnosis conversationally, often telling long, involved stories about situations that paralleled something in the patient's life. He perfected the use of therapeutic metaphor. He made creative use of language with analogies, double meanings, puns, rhymes, guided memories, and humor.

His popularity and reputation followed him into semi-retirement in Phoenix, Arizona, where he saw private patients. Infirm and confined to a wheelchair with arthritis and the recurrence of childhood polio, Erickson held small training seminars in his home for doctors, graduate students, and mental health practitioners until his death.

Erickson was widely revered for the changes he inspired in countless lives. He professionalized hypnotherapy, establishing the American Society for Clinical Hypnosis in 1957 and publishing the first professional journals and monographs on therapeutic hypnosis. Today, the Milton H. Erickson Foundation continues his work through conferences, symposia, publications, and training programs. Erickson helped hypnotherapy gain wider acceptance as a clinical specialty.

Dave Elman was probably the best-known spokesperson for traditional hypnotherapy in the twentieth century. He wrote a leading book for practitioners, aptly titled *Hypnotherapy*.[2] Elman was not a clinician, yet during his lifetime he was a highly influential force in medical hypnosis. He became interested in hypnosis as a teenager, when his father was suffering from terminal cancer. His father's friend, a stage hypnotist, visited the Elman home and used hypnosis to alleviate the father's pain. Elman read avidly about hypnosis and practiced on friends and family.

Elman began his career as a songwriter, performer, radio host, and producer for the Columbia Broadcasting System. Occasionally, he performed hypnosis demonstrations for groups. Several doctors saw him perform and asked him to teach them hypnosis. Elman created a course in medical hypnosis for physicians and dentists. Teaching that course eventually became his full-time occupation.

Elman was recognized for his rapid inductions, no-nonsense approach, and hypnoanalysis, in which an individual is regressed to find the underlying, psychological roots of neuroses and psychosomatic illnesses. He was best known for his method of trance induction, which relied on eye closure. Elman taught that all hypnosis is really self-hypnosis and a hypnotherapist merely facilitates the patient's own trance-work.

Like Erickson, Elman did much to convince physicians that clinical hypnosis could make a contribution to the medical field. He also taught his audiences the value of self-hypnosis for pain management, stuttering, obesity, phobias and fears, allergies, and depression. His work remains an inspiration to hypnotherapists the world over.

Hypnosis and Hypnotherapy Today

Today, hypnotherapy has wide acceptance in medicine, mental health, and sports thanks to pioneers like Erickson and Elman. Many other outstanding practitioners have followed in their footsteps, continuing to shape the practice of clinical hypnosis and advance the teaching of self-hypnosis. Additionally, with advances in brain imaging, scientists have devoted thousands of studies to examining brain activity during hypnosis, discovering that trance accompanies specific changes in brain activity, while facilitating behavioral change, as well.

Here are a few facts about hypnosis and hypnotherapy:

- Over the past half-century, reputable, licensed physicians, researchers, and mental health practitioners have written thousands of books and articles attesting to the efficacy and utility of hypnosis.

- Credentialing bodies in the U.S. and numerous professional boards throughout the U.K. and Europe maintain high certification standards and codes of conduct for hypnotherapists.

- Many hospitals and health clinics now employ hypnotherapists to teach patients how to manage pain, relax, prepare mentally for surgery, and overcome fears and phobias about medical procedures.

- For over four decades, professional training institutes for hypnotherapy have been established in Europe and the U.S., with recognition by professional associations. Professional hypnotherapy training conferences and seminars are held worldwide to help practitioners stay up-to-date with new applications, tools, and research.

- Numerous studies show that hypnosis is safe. Hypnotized subjects have consistently refused to perform immoral or anti-social acts.

Despite these advances, the general public holds misconceptions about what hypnosis is and how it works. In my own practice, I've found that most clients seeking hypnotherapy have a certain mindset about what hypnosis ought to look like and feel like, mainly because they've been influenced by Hollywood movies. Films do not portray hypnotherapy accurately. Therefore, I do a lot of educating my clients about what hypnosis really is ... and for that discussion, we go on to the next chapter.

CHAPTER 2

What is Hypnosis Exactly?

If you were to read 100 books about hypnosis or interview 100 hypno-therapists, you would probably get 100 different definitions of hypnosis. Sometimes hypnosis is defined as a state and other times as a process. Hypnotherapists employ a range of methods for hypnosis and a variety of criteria for determining that someone is hypnotized. Each practitioner has his or her own biases, beliefs, and theories about human psychology. What I tell you in this book is all about the way *I* understand hypnosis. So please bear with me and keep an open mind if what you've heard or read runs contrary to what you will learn here.

Here is my definition of hypnosis:

> Hypnosis is a communication process for inducing, or bringing about,
> a state of trance, for directing mental activities toward an outcome.

That's it! You might have expected something more complex. Most writers in the field of hypnosis use far more complicated descriptions. While my definition is very simple, it holds these four vital pieces of information:

1. **Hypnosis is a process – a set of actions.** The process is communi-cation with another or with oneself.

2. **Hypnosis is a means to induce trance.** It is not the *only* way to induce trance. Moreover, you don't have to be formally hypnotized to go into trance. Anything that can capture and focus your atten-tion and/or imagination can induce trance. Most of us go into trance spontaneously, several times a day. Trance often accompanies medi-tation, prayer, listening to music, romantic encounters, and watch-ing movies or television. If you've ever been "lost in thought," you've been in trance!

3. **Trance is a state.** This means that trance is a mind–body experi-ence. It is not just a thought process, a feeling, or a behavior. Trance

can involve thinking, perceptions, emotions, behaviors, and physical responses, all at the same time.

4. **Hypnosis is a means of directing mental activities toward an outcome.** Trance brings about neurological and cognitive changes. Brain activity slows down. The brain's attentional mechanisms are enhanced, promoting concentration and suggestibility. Trance integrates the parts of the brain involved with problem-solving, motivation, and learning. Hypnosis calms the mind and directs mental activities (such as internal conversation and visualization) toward specific outcomes.

So now let's turn to the subject of trance because it is, after all, central to hypnosis.

What is Trance?

Imagine standing about chest-deep in a swimming pool. You clearly see and hear everything around you. You can wave your arms and talk. Now suppose you duck underwater. It's different. You see people and objects through a watery translucence. It's quieter because water muffles sound. Movement is different too – slower because of the water's resistance. Your body feels buoyant. The difference between standing up and ducking underwater is similar to the difference between alertness and trance.

Trance, for many people, is accompanied by a sense of downward movement. Thus we say that trance can be "deepened." Trance can often change perception. Anything external to self and external to the activity at hand can seem muted – less relevant to the moment. Trance is often said to be a way of connecting with the "unconscious" – that part of being and knowing which seems to operate below the surface of conscious awareness.

The trance state is ideal for relaxation, meditation, intuitive insight, creativity, and accelerated learning. When combined with imagination, trance helps people to visualize goals. Those who don't know much about hypnosis sometimes think of trance as some zombie-like or "knocked out" state or a condition in which one feels weird and spacey. These ideas are highly inaccurate.

Conversely, people who are familiar with hypnosis often describe trance as state of suggestibility, concentration, and/or relaxation. These definitions are *all* correct because all are elements of hypnotic trance.

Levels of Trance

Trance varies from light to deep. Highly hypnotizable people seem to reach deep trance more often and easily than those who are less hypnotizable. Hypnotherapists generally judge depth of trance by two means: (1) the hypnotic phenomena they can observe or elicit while an individual is hypnotized and (2) the hypnotic effects that people report immediately following hypnosis.

With a client in trance, a hypnotherapist might observe facial relaxation, eyelid flutter, or rapid eye movements. The hypnotherapist might also test depth of trance by eliciting behaviors that often occur in response to hypnotic suggestion. Arm levitation, eyelid closure (inability to open the eyelids), and sensations of warmth, coolness, or numbness are common examples. Immediately following hypnosis, clients often report time distortion (they lose track of the passage of time while in trance) and "spontaneous amnesia" (they have only partial memory or no memory of what they heard while in trance) as indicators of trance depth.

There are no hard and fast rules as to what exactly constitutes a light trance or a deep trance. The most common means of explaining depth of trance is to describe what happens when hypnosis is used in conjunction with relaxation. As relaxation increases, trance goes deeper. While hypnotic responses vary from individual to individual, Table 1 shows how people generally experience each level of trance, when relaxation is the means of inducing trance. However, your own experience may differ.

I've encountered many lay people, and a few hypnotherapists, who believe trance must always be deep for hypnosis to be effective. I don't accept that premise. To my thinking, the level of trance that works best depends on the intended outcome and the level of trance with which the individual is comfortable.

Table 1 Levels of Trance

Level of Trance	Description
Awake and alert	You are awake, alert, interacting with the environment. Your conscious mind is fully engaged.
Light trance	This is a state of curiosity and/or concentration. You might feel calm. Irrelevant, external distractions are easily ignored. Your focus narrows. You might find it easier to access memories and images. You remain aware of your surroundings. You retain conscious control over your actions. Some people experience light trance and afterward swear they were not hypnotized because they were expecting something more strange or unusual.
Medium trance	You feel more relaxed. You might feel as though your body is floating or drifting. Concentration is keenly focused. It may be easier, at this level, to think creatively, make new associations, imagine, visualize, entertain new possibilities, and obtain insight. You remain aware of your surroundings, although you may lose track of time. You may or may not notice that you feel more compliant and suggestible. You *don't* feel weird or spacey or zoned out.
Deep trance	Your body feels heavy due to a hypnotic phenomenon called catalepsy (reduced muscle movement as the body prepares for sleep). You may be so absorbed in thought that you are not aware of any physical sensations. Any pain is significantly reduced. You might enter that twilight stage between waking and sleeping known as "hypnogognia."
Sleep	You are in a light or deep sleep.

In my opinion, if the outcome is to learn new behaviors and problem-solving strategies, then a certain amount of conscious, cognitive activity is required: a light trance is probably best. On the other hand, for influencing autonomic processes, such as sleep patterns, blood pressure, healing, or pain, then I prefer to use a deeper trance, if possible. Some hypnotherapists simply trust that the unconscious mind, like an ally, will guide the mind and body to whatever level of trance is suitable for the purpose at hand.

Many clients ask me to "put" them into deep trance because they believe that only a deep trance that will solve their problem. Maybe so, maybe not. Many people get fine results with light or medium trance. Ultimate responsibility for depth of trance does not rest with the hypnotherapist. I usually say, "I can *tell* you to go into deep trance, but it's not up to me. How deep you go into trance is up to you, based on your ability to follow my instructions with an open mind."

Light or medium trance usually works well for self-hypnosis, since these levels allow the ability to direct and monitor your own inner process. Deep trance, however, is ideal as a prelude to sleep. Your level of trance may vary from day to day.

As you acquire experience with self-hypnosis, you'll recognize your own varying levels of trance. Don't worry about whether your trance is "deep enough," because many people accomplish good results even with light trance. Even if you think you are not highly hypnotizable, know that your skill will improve with practice.

By the way, you should know that hypnosis is only one way to achieve trance. Anything that can capture attention and imagination holds the potential to induce trance. Trance is common to everyday experience.

The Unconscious Mind

Hypnosis is regarded as a means of influencing the unconscious. After all, if a person wants to change a behavior, and can't seem to do it through conscious effort, then it makes sense that the blockage exists in the unconscious. The key to success, then, would be to convince the unconscious. But you may be wondering, "What is the unconscious?"

The unconscious has two components. The first consists of biochemical information exchanges and involuntary physical processes that take place outside of conscious awareness. These processes, such as the immune response, are influenced by thoughts and emotions, even though we are not aware it. The communication between the mind and the body is unconscious. The second component of the unconscious consists of neurological processes and information structures that rise to awareness, but over which we have little cognitive control. Examples include obsessions, compulsions, impulses, mental blocks, runaway emotions, dreams, traumatic flashbacks, and deeply engrained habits. Insight, creativity, and intuition also seem to have some elements of unconscious neurological activity.

Self-hypnosis affords the opportunity to influence biochemical and involuntary physical processes through the imagination. Self-hypnosis also changes problematic thought patterns, troublesome emotional responses, and unwanted behaviors through calming brain activity, increasing suggestibility, and training the mind in new strategies. Additionally, self-hypnosis facilitates insight, creativity, and intuition.

Hypnosis and the Brain

Studies with brain scanning instruments show that hypnosis has real effects on the brain.[3] The most consistent finding of these studies is that the brain slows down its electromagnetic activity in trance. This means that, under hypnosis, the brain operates at lower energy levels or electronic frequencies.

During normal wakefulness, the brain runs on 14 to 40 Hertz – the beta frequency. In trance, the brain slips into alpha (8 to 14 Hz – light trance) and theta (4 to 8 Hz – deep trance). The lowest frequency, delta (0.5 to 4 Hz), brings sleep. With this information, we know that hypnotic trance is not something people imagine or pretend.

Hypnosis brings about behavioral change because when brain activity slows, information held in dense neural patterns is less tightly bound. This means that thinking is less rigid and suggestibility increases. Hypnosis also directs brain activity away from the brain's pain receptors, so people naturally feel less pain while in trance. Lower brain frequencies activate centers in the neocortex that allow for attention and focus, so concentration is improved. The relaxation achieved in trance directs energy away from the brain's emotional centers in the limbic region (the midbrain), and allows more activity in the neocortex where reasoning and imagination take place. Additionally, hypnosis seems to strengthen the frontal cortex – the brain's "executive function" – giving more control over motivation, self-discipline, and decision-making. So, you see, trance primes the brain for accelerated learning.

When Hypnosis Doesn't Work

I once had a client who was terrified of flying insects. In warm weather she was afraid to go outdoors because she might encounter bees, wasps, cicadas – you name it. Her fear was apparently not related to any trauma. Her phobia seemed to have begun as a caution that intensified with time. I hypnotized her with the instruction that whenever she went outside and encountered a flying insect, she would remain calm and simply walk away.

She came back a couple of weeks later. I asked her how she was doing with the insect problem. "Well, I'm very disappointed," she said.

"Oh, the hypnosis was not effective then?"

"Well, now when I go outside and see a flying insect, I'm not scared at all."

I felt confused. "Well, then, isn't that what you wanted? It seems that hypnosis *did* work for you, after all."

"Well, yes, it did. But, last week a wasp came into the house and I freaked out!"

You see, to me, a bug is a bug, no matter where it is, but to her, a bug in the house was not the same as one in the yard! A flying bug in the house was still scary! Why? It was because I had said only that she would feel calm about insects that were outdoors. Her mind took that suggestion literally. Even though some people would have automatically generalized the instructions to include insects in the house, she didn't. I didn't antici-pate an insect in her house. I conducted another hypnotherapy session to make sure she could cope with flying insects indoors as well as outdoors. She was pleased with the result.

On another occasion I recorded a relaxation CD for a man who had fre-quent panic episodes. He returned the next week and said he had listened to the CD every night for a week. The hypnosis just didn't work. He was still having panic episodes. I asked what he did while listening to the CD. He said, "While I'm listening, I am telling myself over and over, 'This is silly. This won't work. I'm a failure. This can't possibly help me.'"

Is it any wonder that he didn't get favorable results? I explained that hypnosis is a cooperative endeavor. One purpose of hypnosis is to *replace* negative self-talk, not battle against it. I told him to listen to the CD for another week, and this time, mentally agree with everything I said. He came back the next week to report that everything was fine. He was no longer having panic episodes!

The moral of these two stories: first, sometimes hypnosis doesn't work because the suggestions are too context-specific. The remedy is to visualize and mentally rehearse a new behavior in all possible contexts where you might want it. Second, hypnosis won't work with a negative attitude. The remedy here is to maintain a positive attitude and optimistic expectations about getting the results you want.

These two problems are rare. If I could identify the *main* reason why hypnosis doesn't always work, it would be *internal conflict*. People who have the most success with hypnosis (or any other self-help method) are highly congruent about what they want to accomplish. Hypnosis mostly works to the extent that people want it to work. An unmotivated person will not be persuaded by hypnosis.

Someone, somewhere, reading this book will be saying, "But that's my problem! I know what I want, but I just don't feel motivated to do it!" Let me take care of that problem right now. Believe, me, I've heard it ad nauseam. The world is filled with people who aren't very good at motivating themselves, because they let their negative thinking take over. They want one thing, but they tell themselves something else. So they feel conflicted and incongruent. Here are the most common examples:

- Wanting result A and B, but they are mutually incompatible. You can have one or the other, but not both.

- Wanting the result, but not the work or tradeoffs required to achieve it.

- Wanting the result, but not the attendant problems and/or responsibilities that might come with the accomplishment.

- Wanting the goal, but feeling blocked by fears, inhibitions, and limiting beliefs rooted in past experiences. Your mind is clinging to the past and preventing what you want in the future.

To complicate matters, conflicts often reside in the unconscious and are not available for conscious analysis. Such internal conflicts often spur irrational anxiety, procrastination, and/or self-sabotage. Sometimes it takes soul-searching and brutal honesty to get to the heart of the matter. Some conflicts are negotiable and some aren't. Self-hypnosis is ineffective when you harbor conflicts about what you want to accomplish.

Get very clear about your goals for self-hypnosis. Honestly scrutinize your motives. Acknowledge any fears, worries, or concerns and bring them into the open. That's the only way to negotiate conflicts and make congruent decisions about the outcome.

Achieving insight and reaching resolution on your own takes effort. A clinical hypnotherapist can help you identify your conflicts, work through them, and proceed confidently toward the goal.

Hypnotizability: Do You Have It?

Hypnotizability is the ability to go into trance at will. As a human trait, it seems to be "normally distributed" throughout the population. Statistically, this means that a small percentage of people, about 10 percent, are highly hypnotizable. They seem to have a natural, inborn ability to go into trance. There are also a small percentage of people for whom accessing trance (at least on purpose or at someone's instruction) is extremely difficult. The remainder of the population, about 80 percent, is average. Thus, hypnotizability varies just like other traits, such as intelligence or height. The good news is that nearly everyone and anyone can be hypnotized!

What makes for hypnotizability? Medical hypnotherapist Steven Gurgevich noted that specific psychological factors are generally associated with high hypnotizability.[4] They are:

- The ability to follow instructions.
- A capacity for deep concentration.
- A good imagination.
- An open mind.
- The ability to think non-analytically.
- An interest in how the mind works.

It's a misconception that hypnotizability is linked to mental weakness or gullibility. Actually, the opposite is true. Brainy people are often good candidates for hypnosis. I recall one client who was a member of MENSA (an organization for people with genius IQs). He said, "I want to be hypnotized, but I doubt that I can be – I think my intelligence will prevent it." I simply said, "Well, let's explore that." He turned out to be one of the most hypnotizable individuals I've ever met!

Is hypnotizability innate? Maybe. One study examined hypnotizability in identical twins and found a strong genetic component.[5] However, not to worry – there is also evidence that hypnotizability improves with training and practice.[6] Some are born with it and some develop it.

A few situational factors influence hypnotizability, such as rapport and comfort with the person conducting hypnosis. Even though you want to be hypnotized, if the practitioner working with you doesn't seem completely trustworthy, sincere, or skilled, then you may find it difficult to relax and cooperate. In self-hypnosis, no one else is hypnotizing you, so rapport is not a problem.

By the way, if you've previously tried hypnotherapy and the practitioner told you that you couldn't be hypnotized, get a second opinion. Some practitioners just don't have the flexibility to work with every individual. I've met two people whom I could not hypnotize. One client clearly did not want to be in my office. She had been coerced by a family member and was in no mood to cooperate! I sent her away before the first session was over, without charging a fee. The second client was an older person, who, I'm guessing, did not like being told what to do by someone younger. I referred her on to an older hypnotherapist and she did quite well with hypnosis.

I've had a couple of clients who were told by other practitioners that they were not hypnotizable. After interviewing each person, I found a method of hypnosis that worked uniquely well for him or her. Both achieved satisfactory results with hypnotherapy.

Mapping the Mind

Hypnosis is a method for influencing the mind and changing neurological structures at the same time. Each time you learn something new or change the way you think about something, your brain makes a change. Scientists can study the brain by looking at neurons under microscopes. They can watch brain activity through brain scanning instruments. They can dissect brains and discover their components.

Scientists can see and map the brain because it is physical. We cannot *see* the mind. How can we work with the mind, if we can't see it? How do we describe the working components of the mind? How do we map belief? How do we define the internal processes of decision-making, problem-solving, or creativity? Well, for that, we turn to NLP. NLP provides the concepts that help us map the invisible territory of the mind.

CHAPTER 3

An Overview of NLP

NLP began in the 1970s when Richard Bandler and John Grinder modeled the language patterns of superb therapists, distilling reliable strategies for behavioral change. Today, NLP enjoys a wide following through international conferences, seminars, training institutes, books, and recordings. NLP practitioners work in a variety of fields, most notably in psychotherapy and life coaching. NLP can also be found in sports psychology, leadership training, executive coaching, marketing, sales, advertising, and business management.

NLP behavioral change strategies are ideally suited to self-hypnosis. Most of the self-hypnosis methods in Part II rely on NLP processes and have been adapted from ideas and templates developed by leading NLP trainers, practitioners, and authors. For that reason, I've devoted this chapter to NLP to help you understand what it is and its contributions to the field of psychology – especially in therapeutic change and performance improvement.

What is Neuro-Linguistic Programming?

The name, neuro-linguistic programming is, in some respects, an unfortunate choice, because many uninformed people associate it with computer programming. The original analogy, of course, was that the brain is like a computer. Bandler and Grinder thought of neurological structures as similar to computer hardware and mental processes as analogous to computer software. They studied the way people think and developed strategies to "program" the brain, by influencing thought patterns. While the computer analogy makes sense, the term "programming" has been off-putting to some because it sounds mechanistic.

Definitions of NLP abound in the literature. To complicate matters, over the years, many practitioners, in hopes of marketing to businesses, have dropped NLP's emphasis on trance-work, visualization, and therapeutic change, in favor of teaching NLP only as a communication method for persuasion and influence. In fact, it is much more than a communication method.

Moreover, some NLP practitioners in coaching and counseling advertise that they practice "NLP *and* hypnosis" as though these processes were separate, when, in fact, they overlap. People can't learn new thought processes unless they mentally practice those processes – and that requires an inward focus, which is the essence of hypnotic trance.

Unfortunately, at least in the U.S., NLP is still not a household word, even decades after its inception. The name doesn't conjure up a specific idea in most people's minds. Many non-practitioners who think they know about NLP really understand only a small portion of what NLP has to offer. Moreover, I'm sad to say, some NLP practitioners have done away with the term altogether in favor of branding their own niche in an overcrowded self-help market. Nevertheless, they are usually practicing some aspect of NLP.

To clarify what NLP means, here is a breakdown of each component in the name:

- **Neuro** refers to the human neurological system. NLP is based on the idea that we experience the world through our senses and translate sensory information into cognitive processes. Thoughts affect the body, emotions, and behavior.

- **Linguistic** refers to the fact that we use various forms of communication to understand the world around us and to share those understandings with others. We translate experience into the language of the mind: sounds, words, images, and feelings.

- **Programming** refers to the processes by which we internally code and represent experience. Personal programming consists of internal visual and auditory processes called strategies (thinking patterns) with which people make decisions, solve problems, learn, evaluate, and get results.

In general, then, NLP is the study of internal, subjective experience, and how people order that experience to produce behavioral outcomes. This will become increasingly clear as this chapter progresses.

NLP is Process-Oriented

NLP promotes three values:

1. **Congruence:** the absence of internal conflict.

2. **Choice:** the ability to consider and select the options that exist in any given situation.

3. **Behavioral flexibility:** the capacity to adapt to changing circumstances.

NLP is not based on a theory of "why people do what they do." Instead, NLP is process-oriented. By this, I mean that NLP is about *how* people learn and change. NLP began as the idea of investigating and *modeling* the internal processes with which people achieve specific, behavioral outcomes. The developers found that they could bring about cognitive and behavioral changes in themselves and others by (1) interrupting existing dysfunctional thought processes and (2) replacing those existing thought processes with new thought processes that create more satisfying outcomes.

One example is the NLP process called Visual-Kinesthetic Dissociation, which is useful for alleviating phobias. Bandler and Grinder discovered that phobics use a specific way of thinking about the object of their fears. If, for example, a phobic is inordinately afraid of snakes, he will generally visualize a snake as large, close-up, and ready to strike in slow motion at HIM! He might hear a loud scream in his mind at the same time. If he has had a bad encounter with a snake, he will play the encounter over and over again in his mind, often in an endless loop, mentally reliving the awful moment. The accompanying emotion is intense, overwhelming fear. Conversely, a person who *isn't* phobic of snakes will calmly visualize a snake at a distance, minding its own business.

So, for a snake phobia, the NLP practitioner, using Visual-Kinesthetic Dissociation, will first help the phobic client reach a calm, relaxed state. Then the practitioner will instruct the client to imagine watching a movie of himself in a past encounter with a snake, running the movie forward and backward in fast motion; faster and faster until the image of the past encounter is no longer recognizable. The process breaks up the phobic's usual method of thinking about a snake and dismantles the phobic response.

NLP patterns direct attention away from problematic responses and toward solution-oriented responses. NLP practitioners guide their clients through step-by-step learning processes that often combine trance-work, visualization, eye movements, body movement, breathing, and postural changes. A single NLP process can take from ten minutes to two hours. Most practitioners work in 45-minute to 60-minute sessions. NLP methods are applicable for individuals, groups, children, and adults.

Four Reasons Why NLP is Useful in Behavioral Change

NLP doesn't just tell people to do something different. NLP is a proven approach to behavioral change that helps people remap the mind and program the brain. NLP teaches people the actual *mental strategies* of behavioral change, as step-by-step processes that make effective use of human imagination. You'll be learning many NLP strategies in Part II. The sections below describe four things you should know about NLP in order to understand the rationale behind those strategies.

Reason 1: NLP tells us that people make representations of experience

Bandler and Grinder made it clear that people do not operate on the basis of objective, material "reality." Instead, we operate on the basis of our perceptions. Our perceptions become "mental maps." With our mental maps, we "re-present" the world as we think it is. Our internal representations correspond to our senses: visual, auditory, kinesthetic, olfactory, and gustatory. In other words, our inner worlds hold virtual sights, sounds, sensations, smells, and tastes. We mentally replicate experience. Every representation is enveloped in meaning, through memory and association.

Our maps are always flawed, but they can be improved. The structure of internal experience varies from person to person. The structure determines our thought patterns, meanings, values, beliefs, emotions, and behaviors. When we purposely change the structure of internal representations, we also change related thought patterns, meanings, values, beliefs, emotions, and behaviors. The reverse is also true. When we purposely change our cognitions or learn new behaviors, our internal representations automatically change accordingly. We can reinforce behavioral change through practice and repetition. We can practice new responses in two ways: mentally and behaviorally.

Reason 2: NLP offers simple methods to change patterns of thinking

Do you agree that by changing your thinking, you could thereby change unwanted behaviors and emotions, replacing them with something more desirable? Changing a cognitive process may seem a daunting task, but NLP makes it easy. NLP does it overtly by changing thought sequences called "strategies," and by changing the internal representations that make up those strategies.

Strategies are the step-by-step internal thought sequences that lead to a specific behavior. It is difficult for most of us to describe our strategies in detail because they tend to be unconscious. They are so streamlined, they take place in microseconds. Nevertheless, you don't have to know your strategies in order to change them. All you have to do is alter some aspect of an existing strategy or replace an existing strategy with something more effective.

Another way to change behavior is to change the internal representations that support unwanted behaviors. Representations are the words, images, and kinesthetic components of internal strategies. The best way to do this is through "submodalities." Submodalities are the elemental qualities of internal representations.[7] Submodalities are like an embedded code that further refines our thoughts, emotions, meanings, and behaviors. They are the subjectively perceived characteristics of our visual, auditory, kinesthetic, olfactory, and gustatory representations:

- Visual submodalities include location in the visual field, visual clarity, dimensionality, brightness, color, observed movement, etc.

- Auditory submodalities refer to volume, tempo, pitch, location of origin, rhythm, etc.

- Kinesthetic submodalities refer to temperature, texture, movement, speed, pressure, balance, orientation in space, intensity of pain, etc., and all the visceral sensations that we associate with emotions.

- Olfactory submodalities refer to the elements of smell such as sweet, pungent, fresh, fragrant, etc.

- Gustatory submodalities refer to the elements of taste such as sweet, sour, spicy, salty, and bland, and food textures such as creamy or crunchy.

Two visual representations with the same content could hold separate meanings because of their submodality differences. One could appear close, bright, and three-dimensional. The other could appear distant, dim, and flat. Each representation will activate a different neurological response. Each will call forth different thoughts, emotions, and behaviors. By changing the submodalities of any given internal representation, we then change the associated meanings and the subsequent outcomes.

Here's an example. A client told me he'd always carried a deep sadness because he never knew his father. When this client was a baby his father had been killed. He said it was hard to think of his father as a "real person." His internal image of his father was that of a small, black-and-white photo he'd often seen on his mother's dressing table. With his permission, I told him to make the image of the photo life-size and in color. He said the change gave him a good, warm feeling. Then I invited him to visualize the man in the photo as a living, breathing, three-dimensional person, stepping out of the frame. Tears welled up in his eyes. For the first time in his life, he said, he felt a real connection to his father!

There are two special categories of submodalities worth noting: perceptual positions and time lines. These not only alter internal representations, they also modify strategies in dramatic ways.

1. **Perceptual positions** are the perspectives with which we visually represent events. You can visualize an event from your own personal

viewpoint (an "associated" perspective), the viewpoint of an objective observer (a "dissociated" perspective), the standpoint of another person involved in the event, or even from a God-like point of view. Each perceptual position will give a different meaning to the experience you visualize.

2. **Time lines** represent our perceptions of the past, present, and future. They are internal representations that allow us to locate perceived events in the context of time. With time lines, we can mentally revisit a remembered experience and "know" it has already happened. We can construct a possible future event and "know" it hasn't happened yet. Some people describe their time lines using metaphors such as a path, road, stream or river, or maybe a beam of light or energy.

Through the configurations of our time lines, we assign meanings to the general concepts of past, present, and future, as well as to specific events and time spans. We can chart our internal time lines, bringing them into awareness and manipulating them.[8] In this way, we can reconcile and heal painful events of the past, retrieve worthwhile memories, expand our sense of the present, and practice favorable responses to anticipated future events.

With time line processes, you can mentally travel backward in time and comfort a "younger self" through a difficulty that has exerted its effects into your present; in this way, you banish a current-day problem. You can travel backward to the past to revisit moments of triumph, healing, or happiness and bring those resources forward to meet a present-day challenge. You can travel forward on your time line to visualize a future accomplishment, hold a conversation with a "future self," or mentally rehearse a new behavior. You'll learn more about time lines in Chapter 19.

I once had a client who said that she always felt pressured for time, no matter how much she accomplished. She said she felt as though she was on an assembly-line, going from one task to the next, without any breathing space in between. When we charted her time line, we discovered that her past and future were crowding in on her present, making her present seem very narrow and constricted. When I had her "widen" her representation of the present, her demeanor changed visibly. She said she felt much more relaxed and could actually breathe more easily.

Reason 3: NLP teaches people how to access resourceful states

When people engage in unwanted behaviors, it's because they are in an unresourceful mind–body state. When they engage in unwanted habits, it's usually because they are using the habit as a means to reach a resourceful state – to get comfort or relaxation, for instance. Even though many habits, such as overeating or smoking or drinking, do bring about more pleasant states, the price those habits extract is very high. There's a better strategy.

Through a process called "anchoring," NLP teaches the strategies for accessing resourceful states. The idea is simple. Unwanted behaviors and habits usually occur under specific circumstances in which the individual is not in a resourceful state. However, the individual *does* feel resourceful under other circumstances. Jane might feel afraid and timid about public speaking, but feel perfectly confident when cooking a pot roast at home in her own kitchen.

Anchoring teaches people how to transfer a resourceful state from one circumstance into another. For Jane, the key would be to imagine cooking a pot roast – mentally accessing her state of confidence. Then, while still feeling confident, imagine giving a speech. Then she can reinforce the new state with mental practice. In other words, she can practice giving a speech, feeling as confident as when she cooks a pot roast.

Reason 4: NLP defines the well-formed outcome

One reason why people stay mired in unwanted habits and emotions is that they tend to focus on the problem, rather than a solution. NLP offers the "well-formed outcome" as the ideal method for formulating solutions. The well-formed outcome applies the power of intention. Here are the NLP criteria for a well-formed outcome:

1. **State your outcome in the positive.** Say what you want; not what you don't want. If you create outcomes around what you do *not* want, you are focusing on the problem. If you think only of getting rid of what you *don't* want, your unconscious mind will create an image

of the very thing you want to avoid; you'll be unconsciously drawn toward it.

2. **Make your outcomes about the future.** Your outcomes are about what you are going to do now and in the future, regardless of what has happened previously. Although it makes perfect sense that outcomes are about the future, some people continue to dwell on past fears, mistakes, and regrets when it comes to thinking about what they want. You can't change the past, so put your attention and energies on what you can accomplish now.

3. **Make your outcome self-initiated.** Make sure your outcome is something *you* can do, not what you want others to do. If your outcomes are about what you want others to do, you are bound to experience disappointment. Create goals around your own behaviors and capabilities. You cannot control what others will decide. Granted, your outcomes *could* include the steps you will take to influence those around you. Just remember, however, that you cannot control others, so don't base your success on what they do.

4. **State your outcomes in specific terms.** Our brains seem to code outcomes as accomplishable when we get specific about them. Specific outcomes are behaviors that you can visualize and feelings you can describe. Make your outcomes specific by stating when, where, and how often you want them.

5. **State your outcomes without equivocation.** Equivocation is a hedge – it says, "I'm willing to fail" or "I'm not completely sure I want this." Avoid half-hearted statements like, "Well, I guess I kinda want to exercise, once in a while, when I get around to it." Half-hearted statements are not motivating. A well-formed outcome is stated congruently without any hemming and hawing around.

6. **Make your outcomes ecological.** An "ecological" outcome reflects your responsibilities, needs, and values. If you choose an outcome that isn't ecological, it won't feel right. You won't stay with it. You'll sabotage yourself. Don't commit to any outcome until you've checked in with yourself – consulted your inner wisdom and integrity, so to speak, about whether you can truly commit to this course of action. If you feel uncomfortable or conflicted about your outcome, there

is some issue to resolve. It's prudent to look at the risky side of outcomes, as well as the rewards and benefits.

7. **Make your outcome worth going after.** What is the meaning in your outcome? Why does it matter? Identify the values that make your efforts worthwhile and you'll maximize your motivation. Tying your outcome to your values will make your outcome worth the cost, energy, and time you'll devote to it.

The Power of Intention

The well-formed outcome is about acting with intention. To perform any task with a clear intention bestows self-discipline and motivation. Intention is the first step in effective self-hypnosis. Whenever we make a conscious choice or formulate plans for the future, we are stating intentions. When we act on intention, we are acting purposely. What we don't do intentionally, we do by default.

Intention directs attention. Do you give your attention to what you want or to what you don't want? Do you organize your activities around clearly stated intentions or just drift along waiting to see what happens? By acting on intention, your stance is proactive. Without intention, your stance can be only reactive. Our wants and wishes take on vitality when we revise them into intentions. When we wed intentions to values, we can endure difficulty, discomfort, and setbacks. We can proceed with persistence and tenacity. Intentions and values shape our goals. Our goals shape our representations of the future. When the future looks hopeful and promising, we find the energy that fuels accomplishment.

CHAPTER 4

Mind Magic: Affirmation and Visualization

Affirmation and visualization are the two basic "tools" of self-hypnosis. Affirmations constitute the suggestions you will give to yourself in trance. Visualizations will be the pictures you hold in mind. What we repeatedly picture and tell ourselves exerts tremendous influence on health, emotions, and coping skills, especially in self-hypnosis.

Affirmation and visualization rely on the imagination – the source of mind magic. The brain translates every thought into a neurochemical process. The body responds, at the cellular, muscular, and systemic level, to every thought we think. In this chapter you'll learn about the value of affirmations as well as the five most effective forms of visualization used in all forms of hypnosis.

The Art of Affirmation and Autosuggestion

"In every day and every way I am getting better and better." These are the words with which Émile Coué (1857–1926) taught "autosuggestion" – what today we would call "an affirmation." Coué was a French psychologist and pharmacist practicing in Troyes as the world transitioned to the twentieth century. He believed that positive self-talk had beneficial effects on the unconscious mind, activating the body's natural healing capacities.[9]

Coué designed "formulations" of suggestions for his patients. He sat with each patient and instructed him or her to close the eyes. In a low monotone, he spoke authoritatively, describing the individual's increasing health and wellness; giving reassurances about the disappearance of pain, symptoms, anxiety, and self-doubt. His patients lapsed into trance, visualizing changes in their bodies and in their habits of eating, sleeping, and daily activities. Coué said he was planting the seeds of positive ideas in his patients' minds.

Through autosuggestion, he taught his patients to replace "thought of illness" with "thought of cure." According to Coué, the unconscious mind absorbs whatever we repeatedly tell ourselves and translates the message into physical and mental effects. He taught that the mind turns dominant ideas into physical reality in the body.

He believed imagination is more powerful than will, and that the unconscious mind is more powerful than the conscious mind. Coué had a high success rate in treating many illnesses. Today, a century after Coué, affirmations are widely recommended in a variety of self-help books and motivational programs. Hypnotherapists routinely instruct their clients to pair self-initiated suggestions (often in the form of affirmations) with mental rehearsal as a form of post-hypnotic suggestion. You're probably wondering: do affirmations *really* facilitate change?

Psychologist and educator, Harlan Fisher thinks so. In *The Fifteen-Minute Miracle* he described how he developed a structured, practical self-help program based solely on affirmations.[10] The approach is straightforward. Choose a single intention. Around that intention write 75 affirmations. Record the affirmations in your own voice, leaving a pause after each one of sufficient length that when you play back the recorded affirmations, you will repeat each one aloud as you hear it. Listen to, and repeat, your affirmations for 15 minutes a day for 21 days.

Fisher enlisted others to test his method. They kept journals about their progress. Fisher reviewed the journals and compiled the results. In the beginning, most liked the novelty of the method. Others found it awkward and silly. Midway through the program, people had doubts that affirmations would help. They felt reluctant to continue. Many had to work through their own resistance. Some felt uncomfortable and bored with the daily chore.

Nevertheless, as the subjects continued, they noticed gradual changes and increasingly positive feelings. They developed a keener awareness of the meaning of the affirmations, as well as the process itself. During the last four days (days 18–21) many found themselves reviewing painful events of the past with peace and acceptance. All who completed the program reported positive progress toward their intentions.

Affirmations are often used to replace negative self-talk with something more positive. They are helpful reminders for new habits and new ways of thinking. The point of learning about affirmations in this book is that they also make for suitable self-administered hypnotic suggestions.

Here are a few guidelines for devising your own affirmations:

- Make them personal, containing words such as "I," "me," and "my."

- State them in the present tense. Future tense affirmations ("I will ...") imply that changes are not necessary right now.

- State them in the positive. Instead of saying, "I am not worried about the interview," say, "I feel optimistic and confident about the interview."

- Make your affirmations short and easy to remember. "I generally like myself" is better than "I am now achieving the psychological state of self-esteem and personal dignity that is essential to positive mental health."

Some people dislike affirmations because affirmations don't seem "real," and thereby generate feelings of awkwardness, instead of optimism and motivation. If that's the case for you, I can recommend two remedies. First, express your affirmation as a process of steady improvement, rather than as a *fait accompli*. Instead of saying "I feel confident speaking to groups," say "I am gradually feeling more confident in speaking to groups."

A second remedy comes from NLP Trainer, Steve Andreas. In analyzing the influences of affirmations, he cautioned against affirmations that are overblown or too general.[11] He said that we tend to resist and disbelieve affirmations that are not consistent with current reality. In fact, he disagreed with Coué's formula because it's unrealistic to assume that someone could get better every single day. Thus, you could temper your affirmations with a little wiggle-room, expressing them as a general tendency: "I usually feel energetic" might carry more acceptability than "I always feel energetic." Keep these ideas in mind when you encounter affirmations in the self-hypnosis strategies you'll find in Part II.

The Magic of Visualization

Visualization refers to how we represent imagined or remembered experiences and events. Visualization is actually a multisensory representation involving not only sight, but sound, movement, tastes, smells, and body sensations. When we mentally create an event, the body responds, to an extent, as though the event is real in the here and now. Muscles make micro-movements of the actions we imagine. Glands secrete chemicals that match our emotions. Neurotransmitters surge through the body. Blood pressure, pulse, breathing, and heart rate also respond.

I've encountered a few clients who say, "I can't visualize." It's usually the case that they expect their internal imagery to be clear, three-dimensional, and in full color, like a high-definition television image. Internal imagery isn't like that. Your imagery might resemble vague, blurry, ambiguous images that float in and out of focus. You might *sense* the details more than you actually *see* them. I once had a client who insisted he couldn't *see* anything with his eyes closed. In visualization, you are not "seeing" with your eyes. You are constructing mental images. If you can close your eyes and describe how something looks, then you can visualize.

Visualization is helpful for relaxation. For a simple relaxation method, close your eyes and imagine yourself in a pleasant natural setting. Woodlands, beaches, and mountaintops are favorites. You could use such imagery as your own inner sanctuary in which to converse with wisdom figures.

You can project images onto a "mental screen" or, to use a computer analogy, a desktop workspace, within your visual field. If you watch people when they describe their mental imagery with their eyes open, you'll see that they are looking outward, seeing their images in front of their bodies.

Five Types of Visualization

Now let's turn to the five types of visualization most often used in hypnosis. They are releasing imagery, metaphors for mind–body healing, goal imaging, mental rehearsal, and wisdom figures.

Visualization Method 1: Releasing Imagery

Hypnotherapists often begin trance-work with "releasing imagery" – metaphoric imagery for letting go of unwanted behaviors and emotions. Releasing imagery is useful for symbolically releasing fears, anger, hurts, limiting beliefs, pain, and unwanted behaviors. Here is an example.

- Visualize walking through a forest, while gathering up dead, dry sticks and branches. You carry them to a clearing and dump them into a pile. Light the wood with a match. Watch the fire blaze. Write your problems down on pieces of paper. Crumple each piece of paper and toss it into the fire. As the smoke wafts into the sky, it symbolizes that you are releasing your problems. Imagine singing and dancing around the fire to celebrate that you are free of the problems.

You can also use releasing imagery for freeing yourself from difficult emotions tied to past experiences. For example, imagine trauma-based emotions as bundles of old rags that you gather up and toss into a trash bin. Or you might visualize them as suitcases (baggage) that you stow aboard a hot air balloon. Cut the rope that tethers the balloon to the ground. Watch the balloon float away into the stratosphere until it is out of sight, never to be seen again.

Visualization Method 2: Metaphors for Mind–Body Healing

Fifty years ago, few would have predicted that visualization could halt terminal cancer. Yet, in the 1970s, a husband and wife team discovered that cancer patients who visualized healthy outcomes improved their chances of survival. Stephanie Matthews-Simonton, a psychotherapist, and O. Carl Simonton (1942–2009), an oncologist, were program directors at the Cancer Counseling and Research Center in Dallas, Texas. They conducted a four-year study of 159 cancer patients.

The Simontons were acquainted with mounting evidence that mental and emotional states play a significant role in health and sickness. Reviewing intake histories, they noted that psychological stress generally preceded the onset of cancer. They reasoned that if the mind could make the body sick, it could also help to make the body well. They put their theory to the ultimate test in a recovery program developed to extend the life expectancy and quality of life of cancer patients – all diagnosed as "incurable," all given less than a year to live. The goal was to treat the patients' minds as well as their bodies.

Four years later, 63 patients were still alive, with an average of 24.4 months since diagnosis; 14 patients were symptom-free and 12 had tumors that were regressing. Seventy-six percent of the surviving patients reported that they were as active or almost as active as prior to diagnosis. The deceased patients had lived twice as long as expected. What did the Simontons do to get such results?

They chose psychological interventions designed to instill hope and positive expectations. Their program included training in relaxation, exercise, stress management, and pain management, alongside psychological counseling. Patients were advised to set goals, increasing their will to live. Patients practiced "mental imagery" three times a day for six weeks. Mental imagery training was an essential component of the recovery program. Here are the steps the patients followed:

- Enter a deeply relaxed state, with the eyes closed.

- Make a clear statement of a desired outcome.

- Picture the chemotherapy or medication destroying the cancer cells in the body.

- Visualize white blood cells overtaking and defeating any remaining cancer cells. See the cancer cells as "weak and confused." See the white blood cells as strong and aggressive. (Patients imagined their white blood cells with a variety of metaphors: knights on horseback, vicious sharks, and voracious Pac-Men.)

- See the dead cancer cells being flushed out of the body by natural processes. Visualize tumors shrinking.

- Visualize feeling healthy and energetic, surrounded by the love of family and friends. See yourself accomplishing significant future goals.

- Picture an "inner guide" to consult regarding any problems or concerns. (This step taps into unconscious resources.)

- Open your eyes and emerge from relaxation.

The Simontons were among the first to document the positive effects of visualization on health and immune response. Their book, *Getting Well Again*, became a classic in mind-body medicine.[12] In it, they wrote that visualization helped their patients access "a major source of inner strength." Since then, mind–body medicine has burgeoned, with many alternative therapies incorporating some form of visualization. Visualization has been shown to have salutary effects in a wide variety of diseases.

To access the healing power of the imagination, visualize healing processes in your body. Picture your immune system vanquishing invading viruses. See your cells rebuilding healthy tissue. If you aren't familiar with cellular processes, picture your healing with metaphoric symbols. There are no standard metaphors for each type of illness. Use your ingenuity to create images with which you feel comfortable. Add color, sound, and even humorous details. Here are a few examples of generic healing imagery:

- Imagine you are a microscopic engineer going into your body and directing healing processes at the site of an injury. Enter a master control center in the brain – a room filled with dials, levers, gauges, computer screens, and readouts that monitor and regulate body processes. The controls for each organ and system are clearly labeled. Adjust the appropriate mechanisms to facilitate repair and improve specific physical functions. Imagine regulating heart rate, blood pressure, stomach acid, blood sugar, serotonin, etc.

- Envision miniature work crews in the body: carpenters, construction workers, firemen, custodians, surgical teams, an army of Smurfs, or a host of angels. See them cleaning, repairing, directing blood flow, hooking up new connections, and disposing of debris.

- Imagine a cleansing, healing light coursing through the body, circulating around the site of injury, glowing with intensity. Imagine looking at your cells through a microscope and seeing them bathed in this light. See the light moving through the strands of DNA. Zoom out. See this light stimulating processes of repair, healing, and strengthening in various organs and systems. If you don't know what to picture, designate a color for illness and a different color for health. See the light changing the colors of organs and systems.

- Harry Potter fans can envision a benevolent wizard who chants magical incantations and waves a wand over the site of an injury. See the magic taking place – see the site glowing or sparkling, changing colors, size, or shape.

- Pretend you are in the presence of a great healer. This person speaks to you and prays with you. See light coming forth from this person's hands. The healer takes you to a special temple of health and rejuvenation. She sings and passes her hands over you. Visualize energy entering your body and pulsating at the site of injury.

- Imagine traveling through an enchanted forest with a sparkling stream. You follow the stream to a pool of healing waters. You immerse yourself in the waters. The water balances your energies, cleanses your body of toxins, soothes pain, and restores proper function.

For some years, I've enjoyed a small handbook titled *Healing Visualizations* by Gerald Epstein.[13] It describes visualizations (often with anatomical diagrams) for over 90 physical and emotional health issues. Epstein advises readers to perform visualizations daily for three to five minutes, or more often for symptoms that come and go throughout the day, until the symptoms are gone permanently.

If you aren't sure what to visualize, ask your unconscious mind to playfully generate images for you. Just say to yourself, "Show me a picture, in my mind, of the ideal healing metaphor or symbol for this illness." Then go with whatever your imagination presents. End your visualization with an affirmation such as "It is done" or "My healing is complete." Feel gratitude for your body's healing ability. Express thanks to God, angels, healing helpers, or Infinite Consciousness, according to your beliefs.

Visualization Method 3: Goal Imaging

The Simontons found that visualized goals enhance commitment, self-confidence, and optimism. Today, visualizing goals is standard practice in hypnotherapy and self-hypnosis.

Here are the steps:

1. Close your eyes and enter a deeply relaxed state.

2. See yourself in the future, having accomplished the goal.

3. Step into the picture. See it, hear it, and feel the joy of accomplishment.

4. See and hear your friends and family responding positively to your accomplishment.

5. Feel happy and grateful for having reached the goal.

6. Look back over the steps that led to completion. Visualize the milestones.

7. Return your thoughts to the present and look into your future. See the steps leading toward your goal. Decide your next action. Commit to this action.

8. Bring yourself out of relaxation and open your eyes.

What you repeatedly visualize reinforces your intentions. Visualize a future accomplishment. Then look backward (to the present) to imagine the steps involved. You can apply these steps in self-hypnosis to boost motivation and commitment for any significant goal. Even if you don't know all the steps leading to accomplishment, visualize what you can. Your commitment will prime your mind to direct your attention to relevant ideas, connections, guidance, and opportunities that present themselves.

Visualization Method 4: Mental Rehearsal

Mental rehearsal is a visualization method for changing unwanted behaviors, preparing for challenges, and improving physical performance. Change begins when you visualize a new behavior, skill, or habit. With mental repetition and physical practice, the intricacies of new behavior are committed to memory. Then you can automatically activate the new behavior when the opportunity presents itself.

Mental rehearsal creates new neural pathways in the brain and new connections to the motor centers in the body. It lays down the exact circuitry you'll use when you actually demonstrate your new behavior. You can also mentally rehearse emotional states such as patience or confidence.

Each time you mentally rehearse and/or physically practice a new skill you are making stronger neurological connections that modify the body on many levels. Here are five things you can do to make mental rehearsal effective:

- Put your imagery into a real-world context. Imagine where and when you will demonstrate the desired actions and emotions.

- Involve all your senses. Make your imagery seem real. Imagine the movements in real-time (*not* slow motion).

- Include emotions.

- Give significant, positive meaning to your imagery.

- Repeat the process until it brings the results you intend.

Mental rehearsal creates observable changes in the brain. Researchers at the U.S. National Institutes of Health, led by Alvaro Pascual-Leone observed four randomly-assigned groups who participated in a five-day study on playing the piano.[14] Group 1 learned and memorized a specific one-handed, five-finger sequence that they physically practiced for two hours daily. Group 2 played randomly for two hours a day. Group 3 did not physically play the piano, but they observed the instruction and mentally practiced the sequence two hours a day. Group 4 was the control group. They did no piano playing.

At the end of the five days, subjects in Group 1 showed expansion and development of neural networks in a specific area of their brains. Group 3, the mental practice group, showed *the same brain changes*. The other two groups had no such changes. The researchers concluded that mental rehearsal changes neural pathways in the motor cortex, in much the same way as actual practice.

Nowhere has mental rehearsal received more attention than in sports.[15] Top athletes rehearse their skills thousands of times in the mind as well as in physical practice. Mental rehearsal also helps with public speaking, sitting for an interview, auditioning, and stage performance. If you feel shy, it can boost your confidence in meeting new people.

Most people devote far too much time and energy to analyzing and complaining about their shortcomings and weaknesses, and worrying about how poorly they will perform when the time comes. This only creates "anticipatory anxiety." The more you fret about performance, the more likely it is that you *will* perform poorly, even though, paradoxically, you're fretting because you'd like to perform well. The solution is to focus on the behaviors and emotions you *want* to demonstrate instead. Mental rehearsal is easy. Here are the steps:

1. Sit quietly. Close your eyes. Think of a circumstance in which you want to excel.

2. Think about the next time you'll find yourself in that type of circumstance.

3. Designate the emotional state (confidence, patience, empathy, etc.) that will prove optimum for that circumstance. Naming your state gives it viability.

4. Decide what actions you will demonstrate in that circumstance. Describing your outcome gives it viability.

5. Take your thoughts into that future circumstance. Imagine you are there now, demonstrating your outcome. See the environment. Hear the sounds. Feel the resourceful state. Mentally practice the behavior – each step, each moment. Take yourself to the completion of the experience and feel the satisfaction.

6. Return your thoughts to the here and now. Open your eyes.

Mental rehearsal programs your mind and body to achieve your outcome. It is best carried out on a daily basis, when you can sit quietly, free of distractions, and focus your attention. Obviously, mental rehearsal is a form of self-hypnosis.

Visualization Method 5: Wisdom Figures

Visualized wisdom figures help us to access the unconscious mind, tapping into intuition. When you feel stuck, focus on a wisdom figure for guidance. Wisdom figures can be spiritual entities, guardian angels, ancestors, departed loved ones, animals, fictional characters, or historical personages. If you don't know who to invite into your awareness, ask your unconscious mind to surprise you with the ideal being to address your concern. You might feel amazed and amused by the choice. I've witnessed people who spontaneously imagined cartoon characters, childhood pals, and archetypal images.

Ask your question and wait patiently for the answer. In the realm of imagination, the message you receive might not always be a straightforward communication. Your wisdom figure might show you a picture or a symbol. You might feel an involuntary movement or sensation in your body that signifies the message. You might suddenly think of a melody, poem, or bible verse that holds your answer.

The key to success with wisdom figures is not to force the answers. Don't anticipate or analyze. Keep your mind open and curious, *wondering* what the wisdom figure will say or do. Let the guidance emerge spontaneously in your mind. Some people journal about the guidance they receive, as a way to track patterns, symbols, accuracies, and their own interpretations of the process.

If you don't receive an answer immediately, be patient. Sometimes the unconscious mind requires time to incubate the response. On a few occasions when I received no answer upon consulting my "inner guide," I stumbled onto the answer within a few days. I picked up a book that had a helpful passage. I found what I had misplaced. I heard something relevant in a conversation. You could say that my unconscious mind was cueing me about where to look and what to listen for. I could even suppose that a greater consciousness than my own chose these unexpected methods to respond to my request.

Put Affirmations and Visualization to Work in Self-Hypnosis

The affirmation and visualization methods described in this chapter are basic to self-hypnosis. Like trance, they are natural abilities in which we unwittingly engage several times a day. We talk to ourselves. We make movies in our minds.

Positive intentions, well-formed outcomes, affirmations, and visualization carry a legacy of practical success and validation in research. So why doesn't *everyone* systematically apply these tools? My sense is that many people think something so easy, so natural, couldn't possibly bring about such astonishing results! Some people dislike the repetition required and get discouraged when results are slow in coming. Fisher addressed such "resistance" in *The Fifteen-Minute Miracle*.[16]

He invited his readers to visualize themselves as messenger bringing a new message into the subconscious mind. A guard at the gate refuses to allow new information to enter. The guard explains that the new information is not compatible with existing information, and therefore, unacceptable. Nevertheless, the messenger persists, bringing the new message, day after day. Because the subconscious mind responds to repetition, eventually the new message begins to sound familiar. The guard at the gate finally says, "I've heard this information before. You may enter."

CHAPTER 5

Inducing and Deepening Trance

So far, I've told you about the elements of NLP and hypnosis, but I haven't yet told you how to do self-hypnosis. This chapter is a primer on how to hypnotize yourself. Having completed this chapter, you'll be ready to experience hypnosis with the CD included with this book. You'll be ready to go to Part II and learn the self-hypnosis applications that most appeal to you.

A hypnosis session has three parts: a beginning, middle, and end. The parts are called, respectively: induction and deepening, trance-work, and reorientation. Here is a description of each:

- **Induction and deepening:** This is the beginning phase of hypnosis in which trance begins. Depending how "hypnotizable" you are, induction can take place within a few seconds or several minutes. As you become skilled, you can vary the length of time to suit your preferences. During induction, you'll experience mild physical and mental changes as you relax and your brain frequency goes to alpha. A general rule is to close your eyes. You can perform self-hypnosis with your eyes open; it's just easier with the eyes closed. Closing the eyes will enhance concentration on the mental processes that lie ahead.

  Deepening is the use of additional induction or relaxation methods to enhance trance. You'll learn simple ways to go into trance and deepen trance in this chapter and on the accompanying CD.

- **Trance-work:** This is the centerpiece of the hypnotic experience. Trance-work applies mental strategies targeted toward your outcome. It consists of visualization, affirmations, and an inner dialog between the conscious mind and the unconscious mind. In essence, you talk to yourself and run movies in your mind. This stage of self-hypnosis is generally the longest of the three.

- **Reorientation:** This is the return to full alertness. It is alerting yourself and bringing yourself out of trance. You can reorient yourself by opening your eyes, taking a deep breath, looking around, and shifting your posture.

In this chapter, you'll mainly learn about induction, deepening, and reorientation. I will speak briefly about trance-work, but specific applications will be thoroughly covered in Part II. At the end of the chapter, I'll give information on recording your own self-hypnosis sessions, commercial hypnosis recordings, and how to select a hypnotherapist. We begin with general considerations for self-hypnosis.

General Considerations for Self-Hypnosis

Self-hypnosis is a quiet, solitary activity. Familiarize yourself with these guidelines to make your self-hypnosis experience comfortable and rewarding:

- Begin each self-hypnosis session with an intention and a well-formed outcome. Focus on the solution, not the problem. If you don't know the solution, use the trance-work phase to ask your unconscious to show you a direction.

- During self-hypnosis, sit or recline comfortably. You might want to listen to soft music to set the mood. Loosen tight clothing so that you breathe freely. You might do well to remove contact lenses. Dim the lights and/or draw the shades. If the room is not dark enough for you, put an eye pillow on your eyes.

- Choose a quiet environment that is relatively free of distractions and interruptions. It is unsettling to be jarred out of trance by an unexpected disturbance.

- If you are on a restricted time schedule, set a time frame as to how long you want to remain in trance, so that you'll reorient at the appointed time. In trance, some people lose track of time. Others relax to the extent that they fall asleep. You might want to set a timer that reminds you when your session is at an end. Make sure the alarm is not too loud or disturbing.

- Do not practice self-hypnosis, or listen to any hypnosis products, in an environment where you must remain alert to your surroundings. Don't practice self-hypnosis when driving a vehicle, operating potentially dangerous equipment, or when you are directly supervising the activities of others who cannot care for themselves.

- As you learn self-hypnosis, be patient and kind to yourself. Don't berate yourself or dwell on weaknesses. It's my observation that the unconscious mind is least accessible through negative emotions. You cannot possibly get to alpha frequency if you are chastising your efforts.

- How long is an average self-hypnosis session? Rossi and Lippincott studied people who were skilled with self-hypnosis.[17] They found that the average self-hypnosis session lasted about 20 minutes, with a range of 3 to 37 minutes.

- Even in trance, you'll maintain some degree of awareness of your surroundings. You can bring yourself out of trance instantly for any urgent need.

One of the best ways to learn self-hypnosis is to have a trained hypnotherapist guide you through the process until you can do it unassisted. On the CD that accompanies this book, I do just that! Remember, the ability to access trance improves with practice. For best results, always make the process fun, relaxing, and enjoyable.

Induction: Accessing Trance

Essentially, anything that focuses the mind can induce trance. If you are engrossed in a movie, a video game, or an engaging conversation, you might be in an outward-focused trance. If you are lost in thought, you are in an inward-focused trance. An inward-focused trance is best for self-hypnosis because of the need for inner dialog and visualizing. For that reason, most induction methods require that you remove yourself from distractions and close your eyes.

As you acquire familiarity with self-hypnosis, you'll become adept at going into trance readily. Your sessions will become more time-efficient.

You may discover that you are so attuned to conversing with your unconscious that you do it without a formal trance induction. You'll just close your eyes, relax, take a deep breath, and you'll be in trance. You'll fall back on formal methods when you find it initially difficult to relax and concentrate. Induction methods all have two things in common: (1) focusing attention inward on an image, sensation, or idea and (2) physical relaxation.

If you are a beginner with self-hypnosis, experiment with the methods below to discover which ones work best for you. These are certainly not the only methods for inducing trance – there are many others not included here. You'll notice overlap among these methods. You might combine one or more to develop your own variations. Here are six induction methods that I've found are easiest for beginners. For each one, I've included a short script, giving you an idea of how a hypnotherapist might give the instructions. The scripts tell you what to say if you decide to record your self-hypnosis sessions.

Induction Method 1: Eye Roll (less than 30 seconds)

This easy method focuses attention on the contrast between tension and relaxation in the eye muscles. You first look upward to create tension in your eye muscles, and then relax those muscles, allowing the relaxed feeling to continue on down into the body.

- Sit or recline comfortably.

- Roll your eyes upward toward your forehead. Fix your gaze on something near the ceiling, above eye level, straining the eye muscles slightly. You will feel a slight discomfort around the eyes.

- Hold the upward gaze until your eye muscles begin to tire, within 5 to 15 seconds.

- Inhale deeply. Exhale, lower your gaze, close your eyes, and relax your eye muscles.

- Continue to relax, directing the relaxation from your head down to your toes.

- Say silently to yourself: "I feel calm and peaceful" (or something similar).

- Proceed with deepening or trance-work.

Here is a script of how you would say these instructions on a recording:

> Sit or recline comfortably. Keep your eyes open for now. Roll your eyes upward, focusing on some object above your head or a spot on the ceiling. Keep staring upward as the small muscles around your eyes begin to tire. You'll feel a slight discomfort around your eyes. To relieve that discomfort, inhale deeply. As you slowly exhale, lower your gaze, close your eyes, and feel the relief. Relax the muscles around your eyes. Let the relaxation flow down across your body, relaxing all the muscles from head to toe. Say to yourself, "I feel calm and peaceful." Now you are ready to transition to deepening or trance-work.

Induction Method 2: Arm Drop (less than 30 seconds)

In this induction, suddenly making your arm limp, so that it quickly drops, serves as a signal to relax completely and go into trance. Here are the steps:

1. Sit or recline comfortably. Close your eyes.

2. Lift one of your arms, bending the elbow at a 90 degree angle. Keep your wrist and fingers loose and limp.

3. On the count of one, inhale deeply. Exhale and let your body (except for your raised arm) relax.

4. On the count of two, inhale deeply. Exhale and let your body (except for your raised arm) relax even more.

5. One the count of three, inhale deeply. As you exhale, let your arm go completely limp, so that it drops forward and down instantly. At the same instant, have the sensation of dropping down into a much deeper, relaxed state.

6. Say silently to yourself: "I feel calm and peaceful" (or something similar).

7.   Proceed with deepening or trance-work.

A script for this induction might read like this:

> Sit or recline comfortably. Close your eyes. Lift up one arm, bending it at the elbow at a 90 degree angle. Let your hand and fingers get loose and limp. In a moment, I'm going to count from one to three. With each number, inhale deeply and then exhale, letting your body feel much more relaxed. When I reach the number three, instantly drop your arm down, at the same moment that you drop deeply into hypnotic trance.
>
> One, breathe in deeply, and breathe out, feeling more relaxed. Two, breathe in deeply, and breathe out, relaxing even more. Now three, breathe in and as you breathe out, drop your arm, really dropping deep down into hypnotic relaxation. Say to yourself, "I feel calm and peaceful." Now you are ready to transition to deepening or trance-work.

Induction Method 3: Counting (less than 60 seconds)

Counting is a common method for inducing trance. Just count from one to five or from one to ten and relax your body more completely with each number. You'll automatically access a hypnotic state. Although some hypnotherapists count backward, I prefer to count forward. If you listen to recordings by several different hypnotherapists, you'll hear some who count forward and some who count backward. My advice is to maintain flexibility and cooperate with the instructions, regardless of the direction of the counting. Here are the steps:

1.   Sit or recline comfortably. Close your eyes.

2.   Inhale. Picture and mentally say the number one to yourself. Exhale and physically relax. Let the image of the number disappear.

3.   Inhale. Picture and mentally say the number two to yourself. Exhale and relax more. Let the image of the number disappear.

4.   Inhale. Picture and mentally say the number three to yourself. Exhale and let your body feel heavy and limp. Let the image of the number disappear.

5. Inhale. Picture and mentally say the number four to yourself. Exhale and relax more completely, if you can. Let the image of the number disappear.

6. Inhale. Picture and mentally say the number five to yourself. Exhale and relax more completely, if you can. Let the image of the number disappear.

7. Say silently to yourself: "I feel calm and peaceful" (or something similar).

8. Proceed with deepening or trance-work.

Here is a sample script for this induction:

> Sit or recline comfortably. Close your eyes and release all the cares and concerns of the day. I'm going to ask you to picture and say the numbers one to five to yourself. After you picture and say each number in your mind, let the image of that number disappear. As each number fades from your vision, you'll allow your body to relax more completely. Here we go now.
>
> As you inhale, picture the number one in your mind. Say "number one" to yourself. Exhale and physically relax. Let the image of the number one disappear. It's gone. You don't see it in your mind. You feel much more relaxed. Inhale again and picture the number two. Mentally say "number two" to yourself. Exhale and feel much more relaxed now, as you let the image of the number two disappear. Inhale and picture the number three in your mind. Say to yourself "number three." Exhale and let your entire body feel loose and limp. Let the image of the number three fade away. Inhale and picture the number four in your mind. Exhale and relax more completely, more thoroughly. Let the number four fade from your inner vision. Inhale again and see the number five clearly. Exhale and really give in to the relaxed feeling. Let the image of the number five fade away. Say to yourself, "I feel calm and peaceful." Now you are ready to transition your thoughts to deepening or trance-work.

Induction Method 4: Eye Closure (less than 60 seconds)

This classic method suggests that your eyelids feel so relaxed it seems that they don't want to open. Here are the steps:

1. Sit or recline comfortably. Close your eyes.

2. Inhale deeply. Hold the inhale for 3 to 5 seconds. Relax on the exhale. Do this three times. Continue to breathe freely and slowly.

3. Relax all the muscles around your eyelids and through your eyelids. Pretend your eyelids are asleep.

4. Let your eyelids feel heavy. Continue to relax your eyelids and the surrounding muscles. Tell yourself that your eyelids are so heavy, so relaxed, that you cannot open them. Want your eyelids to stay closed.

5. Try, for 2 seconds, to open your eyelids, but at the same time, keep the muscles in your eyelids so relaxed that your eyelids remain closed.

6. Stop trying to open your eyelids and relax all the muscles in and around your face. Let the relaxation from your face flow down into your body.

7. Say silently to yourself: "I feel calm and peaceful" (or something similar).

8. Proceed with deepening or trance-work.

Here is a script for this induction.

> Sit or recline comfortably. Close your eyes. Inhale deeply and hold your breath for 3 seconds. As you exhale, relax. Inhale a second time, holding your breath for 3 seconds. As you exhale, relax more completely. As you inhale a third time, hold your breath for 3 seconds. Exhale and relax more completely, continuing to breathe normally and naturally.
>
> Focus your attention on your eyelids and on all the muscles around your eyes. Relax those muscles so much, it's as though your eyes want to rest closed. Let your eyelids feel soft, drowsy, and heavy. Continue to relax your eyelids and all the muscles around the eyes. Tell yourself that your eyelids are so heavy, so relaxed, that in a moment, when

you try to open them, they will stay closed. Let the muscles in your eyelids and around your eyes relax so much that if you tried to open them, it would seem like just too much effort to even bother with it. Want your eyelids to stay closed. Understand that when your eyelids stay shut it will give you satisfaction to know that you enter hypnotic trance so easily, so effortlessly.

Now try, for 2 seconds, to open your eyelids, but at the same time, keep the muscles in your eyelids so relaxed that your eyelids remain closed. Stop trying now. Relax all the muscles in and around your face. Let your eyelids remain closed. Feel the relaxation around your eyes. Let the relaxation move into all the muscles of your face. Let the relaxation in your facial muscles flow down into your body, all the way down to your toes. Feel every muscle in your body getting relaxed. Say to yourself: "I feel calm and peaceful." Now you are ready to transition your thoughts to deepening or trance-work.

If your eyelids opened, it only means that you didn't have them sufficiently relaxed or that you tried too hard to open them. Repeat the method until you have success.

Induction Method 5: Staircase (less than 5 minutes)

This method is a variation on counting that incorporates what some hypnotherapists refer to as "vertical imagery."[18] Vertical imagery incorporates images such as escalators, staircases, a path down a hillside, a stone thrown into a pond, and so forth. The images reflect the downward sensation of going into trance. In this example, the staircase induction,[19] I've added scripting for imagery of a pleasant, natural setting. Here are the steps:

1. Recline comfortably and close your eyes.

2. Imagine standing at the top of a staircase, with ten steps leading down into a pleasant setting. Your staircase could be indoors or outdoors. It could lead down to a beach, or a garden, or a room full of beautiful artwork and furnishings.

3. Take in the view from the top of the staircase.

4. Count slowly from one to ten. As you say each number, imagine that you take a step down the staircase. Pause with each step and refresh the image of the view. With each step, relax more completely.

5. When you've reached the bottom of the staircase, you could explore the pleasant setting you've been imagining. Bring in visual details, including light, reflection, shadows, perspective, color, fragrances, sounds, movement, and so on.

6. Proceed to deepening or trance-work.

Here is a sample script for this induction:

> Sit or recline comfortably. Imagine standing at the top of a staircase with ten steps leading down to an even deeper, more satisfying state of relaxation. Let this staircase be one of those old, gray, weather-beaten staircases that lead from a dune or a berm down to a beach. Standing at the top of the staircase, you have a panoramic view of the beach and the ocean and the sky. Take in the picture, seeing the golden color of the sand, the blue of the sky, and the colors of the ocean. See the swells moving on the water and the sunlight sparkling on the waves. See the waves as they crash against the shore. Hear the sounds of the waves washing against the shore.
>
> I'm going to count from one to ten. With each number, visualize that you take a step down the staircase. With each number, you relax more and more completely. One. Take the first step. Two. Take the second step, feeling more relaxed. Three. Another step down into relaxation. You feel calm and serene. Four. Take the next step, relaxing more than you thought you could. Feel so peaceful. Five. Really give in to this relaxation. Six. Relaxing deeper now. The beach is closer now. Seven. Relaxing so much, you can smell the salt air. You feel carefree. Eight. Another step down into that relaxation. Nine. Step down again. Much more relaxed. Feeling safe and secure. Ten. You've reached the final step. You step off the staircase.
>
> Feel the texture of the warm sand under your feet and the cool breeze against your skin. The sunlight is bright as it reflects off the sand and the water. Hear the constant ebb and flow of the tide as the waves break against the shore. You see a formation of pelicans gliding by

silently overhead. Notice the little sand plovers running on the sand, with their tiny toothpick legs scurrying to and fro, playing tag with the surf. See the movement and colors of the water, the vast horizon, and the blue sky. You walk, feeling the sand underneath your feet. You see the texture and colors of the sand, dotted with colorful fragments of seashells that have washed up overnight. Take as much time as you wish, walking along this beach, looking at the ocean waves, the sky, and the dunes. Notice every detail. Everything here is beautiful. You feel peaceful and serene. When you are ready, transition your thoughts to deepening or trance-work.

Induction Method 6: Progressive Relaxation (approximately 5 minutes)

For decades, progressive relaxation has been a standard relaxation training method in biofeedback and stress management programs. It is also used extensively in hypnotherapy as a popular trance induction method. While there are variations, the central feature is a sequential focusing on separate sections of the body while relaxing them. Take your time with each section of your body to make sure the muscles are relaxed completely. Here are the steps:

1. Recline comfortably. Close your eyes. Inhale deeply and exhale slowly, three times, feeling more relaxed with each exhale. Continue to breathe freely and slowly.

2. Focus attention on your feet. Relax your feet.

3. Focus attention on your ankles. Relax your ankles.

4. Focus attention on your calves. Relax your calves.

5. Continue focusing on and relaxing each body section: thighs, hips, buttocks, abdomen, back, shoulder blades, shoulders, chest, arms, hands, neck, scalp, and face.

6. Say silently to yourself: "I feel calm, peaceful, and relaxed" (or something similar).

7. Focus on your breathing for a few moments.

8. Proceed to deepening or trance-work.

Here is a script for this method:

> Get into a comfortable position. Take in a long, slow breath. As you slowly exhale, let your eyelids close. Take in a second long, deep breath, and as you slowly exhale, release all the cares and concerns of the day. Take in a third long, deep breath. As you exhale, become aware of sensations and feelings in your body. Continue breathing normally and naturally.
>
> Focus attention on your feet. Let your feet become completely relaxed. Let the relaxation continue into your ankles. From your ankles, move your attention into your calves. Relax all the muscles in your calves. Bring the relaxation into your knees. Feel the relaxation easing into all the muscles of your thighs. Let your legs and feet feel completely relaxed.
>
> Bring the relaxation into your hips, buttocks, and abdomen. By now, the lower half of your body should feel totally relaxed. Let the relaxation flow upward into your spinal column, radiating out into your nervous system and into all the muscles of your back. Feel as though you are sinking right down into the surface on which you are reclining. Let the surface support your body. Bring the relaxation into your shoulder blades and over your shoulders, down into your chest. Relax more completely with each breath that you exhale. It feels good to really give in to this relaxation.
>
> Let the relaxation flow from your shoulders, down into your arms. Send the relaxation into your upper arms, your elbows, your lower arms, your wrists, and your hands. Relax each hand. Let every finger relax. Direct the relaxation into your neck, over your scalp, and down into your forehead. Relax all the muscles of your face. The muscles of your eyelids. The muscles around your eyes. Relax your cheeks, lips, and jaw.
>
> Let your body feel relaxed from head to toe. Let relaxing images drift gently through your mind, with carefree feelings of contentment. If you wish, take a moment now to follow the motions and sensations of your relaxed breathing, breathing freely and easily, in a detached sort of way. Say to yourself, "I feel calm, peaceful, and relaxed." Focus on your breathing. Feel each in-breath and each out-breath. Now you are ready to transition to trance-work.

A variation on this method is to visualize the relaxation gradually moving through your body as a soft, soothing, healing light or a wave of energy. As you relax each section of your body, bless it with health and healing.

Deepening Your Trance

Deepening increases the intensity of trance. With the exception of the eye-roll method (because you'd have to open your eyes) and the arm-drop method (because it might be slightly jarring), you can use any of the trance induction methods above for deepening.

If you are doing trance-work and find that you have trouble staying with it, just stop and go to deepening and then return to trance-work. If something distracts you and brings you out of trance or up to a lighter level of trance than you'd prefer, go back to deepening and continue your trance-work.

In the previous chapter, and in the staircase induction above, I described how to visualize a pleasant place. This type of visualization can also be a deepening method. Many hypnotherapists guide their clients to visualize a beautiful, natural setting prior to trance-work. Visualization engages the brain in the hypnotic process. You could also recall relaxing experiences you've enjoyed, such as reading a novel in front of a crackling fire, stroking your cat, slow dancing in the arms of your love, or relaxing in a hot-tub.

Trance-Work

Trance-work follows induction and deepening. It consists of directing your thoughts, talking to yourself, stating affirmations, and applying the visualization methods you read about in the previous chapter. You'll learn specific trance-work strategies in Part II.

One way to use trance-work is for quick, on-the-spot self-regulation. A common application is to feel calm and relaxed – say when you are in the dentist's chair, meeting someone you want to impress, or when falling asleep.

Here is an easy method (about 60 seconds in length) that I recommend (it has a short induction, brief trance-work, and a reorientation).

1. Sit quietly and comfortably. Close your eyes. If you don't want to close your eyes, just stare at a blank spot on a wall.

2. Count from one to three and let your body relax a bit more with number.

3. Inhale deeply. As you slowly exhale, let a calming, relaxing feeling come over your body. Say to yourself, "I feel calm, peaceful, and relaxed."

4. Inhale deeply a second time. As you slowly exhale, say something encouraging to yourself, such as "I can get through this," or "I'll figure this out."

5. Inhale deeply a third time. As you slowly exhale, decide exactly what you'll do immediately after you reorient yourself. Visualize doing it. Resolve to do it in the way you've visualized it.

6. Reorientation: Quickly count three, two, and one, while bringing yourself back to full alertness. Open your eyes. Take the action you visualized.

Sometimes a quiet moment of on-the-spot self-hypnosis will help you to reach a decision, clarify confusion, capture a memory, or acquire an insight. Just get quiet with yourself and visualize or ask for unconscious guidance. Other on-the-spot applications include pain management and directing blood flow (to warm the hands and feet).

Reorientation: Coming Out of Trance

Reorientation is gently coming out of trance and back to wakeful alertness. If you've counted yourself into trance, count backwards to reorient. If you imagined walking down a staircase, imagine walking back up the staircase. While these reversals aren't absolutely necessary, they seem to give a finishing touch to trance-work. You could also simply open your eyes, take a deep breath, and slowly get reacquainted with your surroundings. Avoid jolting yourself back to full alertness, as it can be momentarily disconcerting and disorienting, if you've been in a deep trance.

Here's what I say to my clients when I count backward for reorientation:

> Now I'm going to count from five to one. As I say each number, you'll become increasingly alert, so that by the time I reach the number one, you'll be wide awake, fully alert, feeling refreshed. Let's begin. Five, now get ready to come up out of trance. Four, you're feeling more alert. Your physical energies are returning. Three, you are returning to full, wakeful alertness. Think about what the room will look like when you open your eyes. Two, take a deep breath and get ready to open your eyes. One, open your eyes now, feeling fully alert once more.

Here is a reorientation script that has no counting:

> Your hypnosis session is complete. Trust that your unconscious mind has absorbed all the necessary information to fulfill your intentions. Trust your capacity to bring your envisioned outcomes into reality. Bring your thoughts back to the here and now. Prepare to return to conscious, wakeful awareness. Feel your energy returning as you become more fully alert. You are coming up out of hypnotic trance. Think about how the room around you will look when you open your eyes. Take a deep breath in. As you breathe out, wiggle your fingers and toes. Open your eyes now feeling fully alert, ready to continue your day.

When you open your eyes, stretch and take a deep breath. Move around a bit. Of course, you would omit reorientation if you are using self-hypnosis for falling asleep.

Recording Your Own Self-Hypnosis Sessions

Recording self-hypnosis instructions is much easier than memorizing them. Invest in a hand-held, audio-digital recorder to record your own self-hypnosis instructions. Using computer software, you can burn your own self-hypnosis instructions to blank, write-only CDs or download them into a media storage device such as an MP3 player or smart phone.

For a trance induction, simply choose any method above. Read the steps aloud into your recorder microphone. Use the scripts I've provided or say something similar. Make it conversational. Use a second induction for deepening, again reading from the script provided, or make up one of your own. Then go on to record the trance-work, selecting a self-hypnosis application from Part II or a visualization process from Chapter 4. Always end each self-hypnosis session with a reorientation.

When you record your sessions, vary the wording for your own needs and preferences. Speak slowly, in a gentle voice. Pause to allow adequate time to process and follow the instructions. Speed up the pace slightly for reorientation. You'll have my example of how to speak hypnotically on the CD that accompanies this book. With experience, you'll develop your own pacing.

Commercial Hypnosis Recordings

Search the Internet and self-help sections of most book stores and music stores, and you'll find a wide range of commercial hypnosis recordings, audio downloads, and CDs. They range in length from 15 to 45 minutes. Some are sold singly and some are sold in sets. Some have a dual track with more than one speaker giving different suggestions. This "dual induction" hypnosis is assumed to induce deeper levels of trance and have more profound effects. I've been unable to find any research to verify the assumption. Nevertheless, these recordings do make for a unique listening experience.

Some hypnosis recordings contain subliminal communications – whispered suggestions in the background. The idea is that while you listen to one soundtrack (usually music, a monolog, or "white noise"), barely audible suggestions on another soundtrack will bypass any resistance in the conscious mind and register at an unconscious level. If a recording contains subliminal suggestions, it will say so on the package or in the advertising material.

You can find commercial hypnosis recordings with healing visualizations and trance-work for almost any illness. Additional mind–body topics include ease of childbirth, smoking cessation, weight reduction, preparation for surgery, improved libido and sexual enjoyment, stress management, and pain management. Popular self-improvement topics include study skills, self-esteem, self-confidence, achieving goals, sales skills, positive attitudes, and resilience.

Some commercial recordings include background music or nature sounds with a "binaural beat." A binaural beat sounds like a flutter in the background. It's a sound effect technology that assists the brain into alpha and theta frequencies. Headphones are recommended for the stereo effects and best results. A binaural beat is completely safe (except possibly for anyone with a seizure disorder).

You can also buy hypnotic music CDs or downloads, with no words, as background music for your own recordings, or to accompany meditation, visualization, and self-hypnosis. Some also contain a binaural beat. These recordings are royalty-free for personal use. They are mostly sold via the Internet. You can listen to short samples of the music on the vendor's website before making your choices.

Working with a Professional Hypnotherapist

If you find self-hypnosis difficult to learn, or if you aren't getting the results you want, consult a professional hypnotherapist, who can teach you one-on-one. You might want a hypnotherapist who will record a customized hypnosis CD specifically for your needs.

If you think hypnosis might help you to resolve anxiety, depression, trauma, or issues of abuse, a phobia, grief, compulsive behaviors, or the after-effects of a highly stressful and emotionally-charged event, consult and work with a hypnotherapist who is also a licensed psychotherapist. Please do not try to resolve such issues on your own.

Some hypnotherapists work with clients over the phone or with live computer-to-computer video transmission. I may be old-fashioned but I think the best hypnotic effects are achieved face-to-face. Most of my clients prefer to meet in the quiet of my office, away from the interruptions and distractions of daily life.

In choosing a professional hypnotherapist, find someone with whom you feel comfortable and compatible. Most practitioners will let you interview them by phone prior to scheduling an appointment. Some will also respond briefly to an email inquiry. Ask about credentials, training, licenses and certifications, fees, appointments, and scheduling arrangements. Ask, "Do you have experience working with a problem like mine?"

Now You have the Basics

With the first five chapters and with listening to the CD, you now have the basic skills and understandings for a positive experience of self-hypnosis. You'll put those skills and understandings into practice in Part II. There, you'll find specific applications of self-hypnosis that address a number of common problems and issues of personal growth and self-improvement. Select the applications that most closely meet your needs and concerns. I think you'll be pleasantly surprised at how easily you can achieve noticeable results!

PART II

Practical Applications in Self-Hypnosis

Now it's time to experience the many applications of self-hypnosis. Part I described the basic hypnotic processes you'll be using in Part II: the well-formed outcome, affirmations, visualization, trance induction, deepening, and reorientation. In Part II, you'll apply trance-work strategies, the step-by-step processes of self-hypnosis, to solve a variety of issues. In each chapter, you'll find a bit of theoretical rationale as well as practical tips for making worthwhile changes in thinking and behavior.

Each self-hypnosis strategy is clearly marked with a chapter subtitle beginning with the words: "Self-Hypnosis." I've outlined each strategy as a series of numbered steps. With very few exceptions, the first step is to induce and deepen trance. To do so, you'll choose an induction and a deepening method from Chapter 5. With few exceptions, the self-hypnosis sessions end with instructions for reorientation. Exact instructions and a script for reorientation can be found, again, in Chapter 5.

Read each self-hypnosis method once through before actually doing it in trance. As I mentioned in Chapter 5, you could record each self-hypnosis strategy you select, using the text as a script. Then you can listen to your recording comfortably, without having to memorize the steps. When recording the steps, speak slowly and in a calm voice. Insert pauses to allow sufficient time to process the instructions in each step. An alternative to recording is to have another person read the steps to you, while you relax and close your eyes.

Although you'll want to take your time with each self-hypnosis strategy, you'll find most can be accomplished in less than 30 minutes. You'll find a definite NLP influence in these pages. Every self-hypnosis procedure in this book is one that I have used in my practice or have found personally useful. Self-hypnosis is not an exact science with hard and fast rules. Feel free to modify any of the self-hypnosis strategies to suit your individual needs and preferences. Once you become adept with self-hypnosis, you can devise your own self-hypnosis strategies, applying the basic ideas from Chapters 4 and 5.

Self-Hypnosis: A Resourceful Self-Image

To get you started, here is a general purpose self-hypnosis application you might enjoy. It's a visualization process for creating a resourceful, capable self-image.[20] The idea behind the strategy is that if you think of yourself as resourceful and capable, then you'll *act* that way. It's a generic strategy for just about any problematic situation. Here are the steps:

1. Go into trance with any induction method of your choice.

2. Visualize an ideal, life-size, three-dimensional, Technicolor image of your ultimate possible self. Project this image out in front of you, in your visual field. Let this image represent your best qualities and strengths. Give the "you" in the image the posture, breathing patterns, facial expression, and movements that convey inner strength and the ability to meet challenges.

   This image has no context. For this other "you" choose any clothing you wish – it could even have a magical look, like a long, flowing robe. You could also surround this other "you" with positive, flowing energy. This other "you" possesses your best qualities and the ability to solve problems and overcome obstacles. Imagine that this other "you" is looking at you with love and compassion.

3. Imagine that your visual field is like a large computer screen – the desktop of your mind. Imagine that this idealized other "you" is a computer file, opened on the desktop. Mentally move an imaginary cursor arrow up to the upper right of this image and click, closing it. See the image shrink into a yellow file icon, moving it to the lower left of your screen.

4. Practice opening and closing the image file, so that you easily visualize it. Move a cursor over the folder. Click on it. Mentally, see it quickly open, moving up toward the right and outward until it fills the screen. Click on the file again to close it. Repeat this process four or five times.

5. Open the file again and visualize the image. This time, watch it transform into a ball of pulsating energy. The ball of energy moves rapidly toward you, carrying useful knowledge and understandings. Imagine that you absorb this energy into your body, so that the energy is downloading information into every cell, into every molecule. Let the qualities of this potential self be imprinted on your DNA. You *are* your ideal self. You have incorporated all this resourcefulness into your being. Feel the transformation taking place within. Imagine the energy surging through your body!

6. Know that you can repeat Step 5 in future situations where you want to feel resourceful and competent.

7. Mental rehearsal: Visualize a challenging future situation. Associate fully into your representation of that situation. See what you would see. Hear what you would hear. In your visual field, see the small yellow file icon. Open the file. See your ideal self. The image instantly transforms into a being of light and energy. The energy surrounds you, downloading into your body. You instantly feel the transformation taking place within. Feeling resourceful and competent, imagine how you'll handle that situation effectively, what you'll say, do, think, and feel.

8. Affirmation: I am a resourceful, competent individual.

9. Return your thoughts to the here and now. Reorient and open your eyes.

A Word about Personal Ecology

For each application you choose in Part II, you are choosing an outcome – a new response. Recall from Chapter 3 that one element of a well-formed outcome is that the new response is ecologically sound. By "ecologically sound," I mean that your outcome matches your internal integrity. You feel free of any conflict concerning the change you anticipate.

I recommend that as you read over each self-hypnosis strategy you select, you check your personal ecology. This means that you carefully examine your thoughts and emotions to make sure you feel completely congruent allowing this change to take place. If so, proceed with the self-hypnosis. If not, ask yourself a few questions:

- Do I anticipate any drawbacks to bringing about this change? If so, what are they?

- Do I feel any reservations or discomfort about having this change? If so, what inner conflict do I need to resolve? Is it possible that some basic need or value seems threatened by this change? In other words, does making this change seem to pose a risk (no matter how slight) to my safety, security, comfort, health, success, enjoyment, friendship, love, identity, worthiness, or capabilities? Is the discomfort telling me something I ought to acknowledge and attend to, before I make this change?

- Do I give myself permission to create this change? If not, what is missing? What stops me? Is there something else I ought to take care first?

Honor the answers you receive. With the answers, you'll get information on how to modify each strategy to meet your needs.

Each time you complete a self-hypnosis strategy, that's another good opportunity to check your ecology again, to make certain you feel congruent with the change. If for any reason you do not feel congruent, ask these three questions again and decide how to modify the strategy to meet your needs. Then, repeat the self-hypnosis session with your own modifications. In respecting your own ecology, the behavioral changes you create through self-hypnosis are far more likely to be consistent and lasting.

CHAPTER 6

Eliminate Unwanted Habits and Addictions

In *First Things First*, published in 1994, motivational author and speaker, Stephen Covey, listed the characteristics of addiction.[21] He culled items from literature on addictions and recovery to compile the list shown below. The first seven items are from Covey; I've added three more. An addiction can be defined as any experience that:

- Temporarily eradicates pain and other unpleasant or negative sensations.

- Creates predictable, reliable sensations that are pleasant, for the moment.

- Becomes one's primary focus and absorbs attention, taking up increasing amounts of time and expense.

- Provides an artificial sense of self-worth, power, control, security, intimacy, or accomplishment.

- Exacerbates the problems and feelings it is supposed to remedy.

- Decreases the ability to function well.

- Damages relationships with loved ones.

- Involves elements of denial and is supported by defense mechanisms.

- Is progressively risky, dangerous, and harmful to self and/or others.

- Always asks for more of itself.

Most of the items on the list apply to unwanted habits as well. We generally think of addictions as involving some substance that enters the body – like a drug. Habits, on the other hand, usually involve repetitive behaviors. Unwanted habits run the gamut from anxiety-reducing behaviors such as nail-biting and hair-pulling to out-and-out compulsions like gambling, shoplifting, pornography, hoarding, self-cutting, and promiscuity.

Negative self-talk, frequent explosive anger, constant texting or video gaming, chronic complaining, and petty arguing also qualify.

Unwanted habits and addictions diminish the quality of life and rob people of the energies with which they could pursue other enriching and fulfilling activities. Habits and addictions rob us of the time and energy to contemplate life's big questions that concern personal integrity, authenticity, values, purpose, meaning, and spirituality. Addictions and harmful habits not only carry risks; they also carry a social stigma of personal weakness, irresponsibility, and poor judgment. No matter how much people defend their habits and addictions, behind the bravado there is often shame, guilt, and impaired self-esteem.

Most people ignore, rationalize, or justify their habits and addictions until problems develop. By then, the habit or addiction seems intractable. Most people cannot "just say no" or "just stop," because the behavior is no longer under voluntary control. It takes on a life of its own. We don't control habits and addictions. They control us.

Habits become intractable because of brain processes that "program" repetitive thoughts, emotions, and actions. Our brains have complex mechanisms for learning and memory. The brain makes automatic anything we do often and frequently. Addictions are difficult to eliminate not only because they entail repetitive behaviors; when addictive substances repeatedly enter the body, the body cells develop additional capacity to accommodate, expect, and eventually *demand* the chemical change brought about by that substance.

Like a muscle, the brain grows stronger in the ways it is used. Neuroscientist Norman Doidge wrote that addictions create long-term changes in the brain, often reaching the point where moderation is impossible.[22] For many, the only solution is complete abstinence. There is good news, however. When habitual behaviors stop, the neural networks supporting that activity shrink as the brain diverts growth to accommodate new behaviors.

This chapter features two NLP processes for conditioning your mind to release habits and addictions. One, the NLP Six-Step Reframe, helps you to define the underlying, unconscious motives that often support unwanted behaviors. The other, Meta-NO/Meta-YES, teaches you to say "NO" to a habit or addiction and "YES" to new, replacement behaviors and rewards. First, however, in the sections that follow, you can assess your readiness for change, followed by a reminder that replacing habits and addictions with new behaviors often ensures success.

Assess Your Level of Readiness

The first step in eliminating deeply entrenched habits and addictions is to decide whether you are really ready to do so. In 1979, James Prochaska, a psychologist, developed the Transtheoretical Model of Change showing that people overcome habits and addictions with varying degrees of readiness and often with ambivalence.[23] His model describes the six stages of readiness that lead to lasting behavioral change. Each step is described below, with tips on how to advance to the next stage. Read through these paragraphs and decide what stage best describes your situation. Then you'll know just how ready you are to release your habit or addiction and what to do next.

1. **Pre-contemplation:** People in pre-contemplation don't intend to take action in the next six months. They may deny that a problem exists, even when others see it clearly. They may attend a therapeutic program at another's insistence, but do not participate wholeheartedly. They lack information about their problem and make no attempt to learn about it. They may resist change because they believe they cannot be helped.

    To advance to the next stage, admit you have a problem. Acknowledge that the methods you've tried, in order to accommodate the problem, control it, hide it, and live with it, aren't working.

2. **Contemplation:** People in contemplation intend to take action within six months. They acknowledge the problem and think seriously about solving it. They want to understand it. Other priorities may prevent them from seeking help.

    To advance to the next stage, obtain information about the problem and methods of treatment. Get information on how others have successfully released the habit or addiction. Resolve other priorities that may interfere with a sincere commitment to behavioral change. Confront any ambivalence and work through it, possibly with the help of a therapist or life coach.

3. **Preparation:** Individuals in this stage intend to take action within the next 30 days and have taken some initial steps. They are developing a plan and making preparation.

   To advance to the next stage, finalize your plan with scheduled milestones. Set concrete goals for observable, verifiable change. Visualize what you'll do differently when you are free of the habit or addiction.

4. **Action:** People in this stage have overtly modified their behavior. Friends and family may notice and give support.

   In this stage, congratulate yourself that you have taken action. The challenge now is to maintain the change. Remember: new behaviors may seem awkward at first, but will gradually become more comfortable and familiar. Bear with the awkwardness. Enlist support from others. Join a support group. Hire a therapist or life coach. Ask her to monitor your progress and hold you accountable for it. She will help you work through the rough spots and surmount unanticipated obstacles.

5. **Maintenance:** People in this stage have maintained behavioral change for more than six months. This is the time to consolidate gains and focus on preventing relapse. Especially with addictions, relapse is the rule rather than the exception.

   To make lasting change, develop a plan for relapse prevention. Identify likely relapse triggers and develop coping strategies that incorporate new responses. Continue to use your support structure, even when it seems you don't need it. If you relapse, don't give up or consider yourself a failure. Relapse contains useful information on how to improve your efforts. Revise, regroup, and start over.

6. **Termination:** Individuals in this stage believe the unwanted behavior will never return and have no fear of relapse.

Eliminating habits and addictions requires that you identify the triggers and circumstances that activated unwanted behaviors. Some you'll want to avoid altogether from now on. For other triggers and circumstances that are unavoidable, decide on new responses and coping mechanisms. For help with coping skills, see Chapter 16.

If negative emotions have triggered your habit or addiction, develop the capacity to perceive negative emotions without the need to act on them. Change begins when you realize that not every thought is a valid thought: it isn't necessary to act on every urge. Relabel intrusive, unwanted thoughts and urgings so that they mean something else. A compulsive eater, for example, might relabel thoughts about food as signaling a need for rest or comfort.

Develop New Habits to Replace Old Ones

When you eliminate one behavior, it may be helpful to replace it with another. You might, for example, have a cup of decaffeinated coffee after supper instead of having dessert. You might want to start manicuring your nails instead of chewing on them. You might want to go to bed on time instead of staying awake to play computer games.

If you have trouble staying with a new behavior, listen carefully to the disparaging thoughts that block motivation, and override them with encouraging self-talk. If the new behavior is a complex one, such as learning a new skill, gradual immersion may be the key to success. In this way, incremental progress allows you to learn as you go along. Starting small often carries less risk of major mistakes and discouragement; you get the reinforcement of small successes, instead of massive failures. Success in almost any major endeavor is achievable in small, doable steps. For more ways to improve motivation, see Chapter 11.

Use self-hypnosis to mentally rehearse new behaviors and to visualize positive outcomes and rewards. Mental rehearsal programs new neurological connections through mental "practice." You can also visualize a role model (i.e., a wisdom figure) carrying out the new behavior and then coaching you on how to do it and stay with it.

Self-Hypnosis: NLP Six-Step Reframing

NLP supports two principles when it comes to eliminating unwanted habits and addictions:

- All behaviors, even problematic ones, are based on underlying positive intentions, usually having to do with satisfying basic needs, such as safety, security, comfort, protection, love, and self-esteem. These positive intentions often lie outside of conscious awareness. Through self-hypnosis, we can access this unconscious material to increase self-understanding and "negotiate" solutions with the unconscious mind.

- Most problematic behaviors originally develop in an attempt to solve a problem. When such behaviors have outlived their usefulness, they can be reprogrammed through new strategies. Habits and addictions are usually behaviors that seemed useful in the beginning, but eventually became a nuisance, having outlived any usefulness.

Bandler and Grinder developed the NLP Six-Step Reframe, based on these two principles, for eliminating unwanted habits and addictions.[24] This pattern is called a "reframe" because it changes the framework with which you think about a problem behavior. It is based on the idea that habits and addictions represent a "part" of the mind that is trying to satisfy a positive intention. However, the "part" has run amuck, generating behavior that is no longer wanted. The idea behind the Six-Step Reframe is to negotiate with the "part" to satisfy the positive intention in another way.

Here is an overview. Visualize the part. Ask the part for its positive intention. Explain to the part that, while the intention is positive and helpful, the resulting behavior is not. Ask the part to access your creativity to find other ways to accomplish the positive intention. Remember, the object is *not* to think of ways to combat urges and cravings. The object is to think of new ways to satisfy the *positive intention*.

This process relies on internal representations: imagery and dialog. You'll converse with your unconscious mind. Approach this process in a playful, spontaneous way, realizing that there are no right or wrong answers. Additionally, I caution you that you must be friendly and kind toward the part. I've had numerous clients approach this exercise with the idea of "punishing" or "getting even" with a part. I assure you that such an attitude just will not work. Your unconscious mind will not cooperate.

The crux of this NLP strategy lies in Step 2 – determining the positive intention. Get this step right and the rest of the steps flow smoothly. Sometimes the positive intention is initially expressed as a *hurtful* intention. The hurtful intention might be something like "to punish you" or "to make you ashamed." If you encounter a hurtful intention, ask again, "What is the positive intention of *that* (i.e., to punish you, make you ashamed). Eventually you'll discover a positive intention.

If the positive intention is vague, ask for more detail. For example, if the positive intention is "Protection," ask "Protection from what?" If the positive intention is "To prevent bad things," ask "What bad things?" This clarification will help with the remaining steps. Here are the steps for the NLP Six-Step Reframe:

1. Go into trance with an induction method of your choice. Visualize the part of yourself that promotes your habit or addiction. See it as a metaphoric image. If you aren't sure what to visualize, ask your unconscious mind to present an image.

2. Welcome that part of yourself and thank it for being available. Ask, "What is the positive intention of this habit (or addiction)?" The answer will emerge intuitively. Keep your mind open and curious as you wait patiently for the answer. Ask for clarification as needed.

    Contemplate the answer. It might be what you expected, or not. It might give an insight into past influences. Self-understanding is a byproduct of this process. Appreciate how your unconscious mind has been trying to work all this out, behind the scenes of your awareness.

3. Appreciate the positive intention. Realize that this part has worked long and hard to satisfy the positive intention, but usually not succeeding. Why? Because the habit or addiction chosen to meet the

intention doesn't work, carries too many risks and disadvantages, or has outlived its usefulness. Talk to the part, explaining how the habit or addiction is hurtful, inappropriate, and wrong.

Ask the part to access your creativity to find suitable alternatives for satisfying the positive intention appropriately. Suggest that there are many options and alternatives. Tell the part to brainstorm new possibilities, select three alternatives, and present them to you within moments. Remind the part that the selections must be doable, realistic, and appropriate. Wait patiently until the part presents three alternative behaviors.

4. Thank the part. Ask it to agree that it will rely on the alternatives whenever it wants to accomplish the positive intention. Remind the part that, should it need additional flexibility in serving your needs, it can, once more, access your creativity and select more alternatives, as long as they are appropriate. When you have this agreement, thank the part.

5. Mental rehearsal: Realize that the habit or addiction is no longer necessary. It serves no purpose. Visualize moments in your future when you are satisfying the positive intention by carrying out the alternatives selected in Step 3.

6. Give yourself the suggestion that whenever you want to accomplish the positive intention, you will pursue alternative one, two, or three. Example: "From now on, when I want to relax at home after work (instead of smoking, overeating, drinking alcohol, etc.), I enjoy taking a walk with my dog, listening to music, or soaking in a hot bubble bath."

7. Return your thoughts to the here and now. Reorient and open your eyes.

Self-Hypnosis: Meta-NO/Meta-YES

Would you like to get very clear about what you want and don't want? Would you like to say "NO!" to habits and addictions and really mean it? Would you like to say "YES!" to healthy living and really mean it? The Meta-NO/Meta-YES strategy provides the mindset of certainty and determination.

The strategy comes from NLP trainer, L. Michael Hall.[25] It helps you to say "NO!" and "YES!" by pairing emotions with statements of refusal or agreement. Instead of saying "no" in a weak, wimpish way, you can say "NO!" in an intense state of refusal! Instead of saying "yes" in a namby-pamby way, you can say "YES!" with enthusiasm and determination! Here are the steps, adapted for self-hypnosis:

1. Induce trance with any method of your choosing. Identify the habit or addiction you no longer want. Set your intention. Express it as a refusal: "I refuse to ..."

2. Access your ability to say "NO!" Mentally review the many ways in which you forcefully say "NO!" to things you don't like or don't want. For example, have you ever scolded an unruly pet with a firm "NO!"? Have you ever stopped someone from doing something harmful, with a loud, firm "NO!"? Have you ever turned down an aggressive sales person with an adamant "NO!"? If someone insisted that you to rob a bank, you'd surely say, "NO!" Get playful with these "NO!'s" Mentally practice saying "NO!" in all the ways you can muster, until you can easily access the feelings that accompany a definite "NO!"

3. Develop a powerful "NO!" state. Mentally review various phrases that convey "NO!" such as: "Never again!" or "No way!" or "Get lost!" or "Listen to me, I said 'NO' and that's final!" or "No, thanks" or "Not today" or "Not on your life!" Mentally practice all kinds of "NO!" statements. Keep going until you are in a "NO way; absolutely NOT; never in a million years" frame of mind. By the end of this step, you'll *feel* a state of total refusal!

4. Condition your "NO!" state. Remember when you recently engaged in the habit or addiction. See yourself about to do it, as a dissociated image. Want to stop yourself! Associate into the image. Say "NO!" in all the ways you practiced it in Step 3. Keep saying "NO!" until you feel a powerful, adamant state of refusal. Repeat this step several times, with remembered instances in which you were just about

to engage in the habit or addiction. Step into each one and say a powerful, effective "NO!" until you absolutely *refuse* to continue the behavior.

5.   Mental rehearsal: Think of future situations that might offer triggers for the habit or addiction. For each one, mentally rehearse saying a forceful "NO!" in several different ways. You are building a powerful "NO!" mindset that you can access automatically whenever you are faced with a situation that was once a trigger. Now you know how to say "NO!" and mean it!

6.   Now that you can refuse that habit or addiction, what do you want to say "YES!" to? Identify two or three new behaviors that will replace the habit or addiction. Imagine what you'll do differently when you encounter the old triggers and environments. Now you are setting a new intention. Express your intention as a statement: "Now I say 'YES!' to …"

7.   Develop a powerful "YES!" state. Review the many ways in which you say "YES!" with enthusiasm and determination. Use your imagination. For example, if someone offered you a large sum of money, no strings attached, what would you say? "YES! Absolutely!" What if your sweetheart asked you for a hug? You'd say, "Sure!" If someone called out your name in a crowd, you'd answer, "Yes, that's me!" If someone asked, "Are you sure one and one equals two?" you would say, "Yes, of course." Get playful and review the various ways in which you can say "YES!" Generate the feelings associated with each "YES!"

8.   Enhance your "YES!" state. Mentally practice the various ways to say "YES!" You've probably had occasion to say "You bet!" or "Yeah!" or "Yes, of course!" Mentally practice all kinds of "YES!" statements – with appropriate feeling, volume, and voice tone. Keep doing this for several moments until you are in a totally convincing "YES!" state.

9.   Mental rehearsal: Visualize your *new* behaviors. Imagine you are right there, right now, saying "YES!" to each one and accessing your powerful "YES!" state. By learning to say "NO!" and "YES!" powerfully, you are taking charge of your choices.

10. Affirmation: When I say "NO!" I mean it. When I say "YES!" I mean it. I firmly say "NO!" to habits and addictions. I enthusiastically say "YES!" to new, healthy behaviors.

11. Return your thoughts to the here and now. Reorient and open your eyes.

Use Your Imagination

Many of my clients have so identified with their habits and addictions that they find it hard to imagine living any other way. They have forgotten what it's like to be a person who doesn't even entertain a thought about the habit or addiction. They think only about struggling *against* the cravings and urges, rather than being free of them altogether. For many people it takes a huge leap of imagination to turn one's thinking around and take on an entirely new aspect of identity.

One step is to stop glorifying the habit or addiction – bragging, for example, about the funny things you did the last time you were high. Stop talking about how much you'll miss it. Stop commiserating with others about how hard it is to give it up. Stop associating with others who are still in the throes of the addiction or habit. Stay away from places and people that you associate with the habit or addiction.

For some people the only way to get free is to hit the wall, so to speak. For a smoker, it might be a diagnosis of cancer. For an overeater, it might be a diagnosis of diabetes. For an alcoholic, it might mean a tragic automobile accident while driving drunk. For a drug addict, it might mean waking up in a hospital emergency room after an overdose. Ask yourself: How far does your habit or addiction have to go before enough is really enough? When can you honestly say, "No more!"?

The NLP Compulsion Blowout may help. You may need an NLP practitioner to guide you through the process, because for many people it is uncomfortable and distasteful – so they bail out too soon, before the process is complete. The key to success is to vividly imagine indulging in your addiction or habit excessively. That would mean, for example, smoking cigarette after cigarette, drinking cocktail after cocktail, or eating cookie after cookie until you feel nauseated. It would mean playing video games hour after hour until you feel exhausted and completely disgusted with yourself.

In a recent study at Carnegie Mellon University, researchers found that people who imagined repeatedly eating a certain food (cheese or candy) subsequently had less desire to eat that food.[26] The researchers attributed the finding to "habituation," which occurs when more of something leads to less desire for that something. The interesting thing about this study is that the habituation occurred in the imagination!

Perhaps you can imagine "over-indulging" to the point where you can stop. Perhaps you can imagine the risks your habit or addiction entails, to the extent that you draw the line, here and now. Perhaps you can imagine the rewards you'll enjoy when you free yourself from an unwanted habit or addiction.

CHAPTER 7

Yes, You *Can* Stop Smoking!

"Of course, the sad part is this. If I stop smoking, I can no longer practice as an attorney. I'll have to give up my career." I stared in confusion at this new client. He was well-groomed and impeccably dressed. Other than the fact that he smoked, he looked to be in good health.

"How do you figure that?" I asked.

"Well, when I go for more than two hours without a cigarette, I can't concentrate, I get nervous and irritable. I could never walk into a courtroom again with those kinds of problems. I can't function without cigarettes."

I couldn't believe my ears! Here was a well-educated, successful man, who smoked 20 cigarettes a day, and had no clue about the facts of nicotine addiction. In his mind, smoking was the *cure* to his ailments, not the *cause*. He'd never stopped smoking long enough to find out that poor concentration and irritability are just the temporary symptoms of nicotine withdrawal. Instead, he thought he would suffer permanent disability! This lawyer, who thoroughly researched every case he ever argued, had never bothered to learn the facts that would make an airtight case against a mass murderer: nicotine.

Smoking is a deadly addiction that kills millions. Smoking is the equivalent of having a life-threatening illness. I don't know about you, but if I had a life-threatening illness, I'd get my hands on information about every treatment ever documented. I'd talk to specialists and those in recovery. I'd get to know the enemy.

People who smoke don't think that way. Like the attorney, they inhale a deadly carcinogen numerous times a day because "it helps me to relax." Yeah – like eating rat poisoning is relaxing! While smokers *know* smoking is hazardous to health, they think, "But that won't happen to me" or "I'll eventually stop before there is any serious damage." So they ignore the facts, remaining in blissful denial.

After all, they reason, smoking is a private decision; an act of free will. "It's not illegal. It doesn't hurt anyone else. What I do with my own body is my business." They ignore statistics about the dangers of second-hand smoke. They don't realize that others resent the butts that smokers leave behind along sidewalks and streets. They don't realize that others are offended by the smell. They dismiss the worried pleadings of friends and loved ones to stop. They don't think about the example they set for their children or grandchildren. They don't know that smokers cost their employers twice as much as non-smokers in insurance premiums, sick leave, disability, and hospitalizations. Do you really think smoking is a *private* decision?

If you think smoking harms no one else, think again. When we hurt ourselves, we hurt those who love us. The diseases that smoking causes are very real and affect not only those who smoke, but their family members as well. My mentor, NLP trainer Ron Klein,[27] once said, "The image I like to use with smokers is that they take themselves into a future in which they did *not* stop smoking. They are lying in a hospital bed with tubes stuck in their body: an oxygen tube in the nose, an intravenous tube in the arm, and they are barely breathing, gasping for air in an oxygen tent. At the foot of the bed, loved ones are standing there, not with sadness, but with anger, thinking 'Why did you put us through this?'"

Smoking is both an addiction and a habit (see Chapter 6). The addiction is to nicotine, an addictive chemical. The habit is the ritual of smoking. A cigarette is the delivery mechanism for nicotine, requiring that the smoker inhale a host of deadly toxins and carcinogens. Nicotine creates a physical dependency as the cells create millions of new receptors to accommodate it. When the nicotine "fix" loses its potency, usually in a few hours, the cells demand more.

Smoking is a leading cause of preventable death. Fortunately, when you stop smoking you can add years to your life expectancy. According to the American Cancer Society, within three months, aerobic capacity increases up to 30 percent. Within nine months, coughing, sinus congestion, fatigue, and shortness of breath decrease. Cilia regrow in the lungs with increased ability to handle mucus. In one year, risk of coronary heart disease is *half* that of a person who smokes.

As more governments pass laws banning smoking from public places, as publicity about the health hazards of smoking increases, and as the cost of cigarettes rise, more people want to stop smoking. Remember, smoking is not your identity; it's a behavior you can change. So get out of the denial and reclaim your lease on life.

Prepare to Stop Smoking

To stop smoking, choose a target date at which time you'll stop smoking. Choose a time frame that won't be too stressful in other ways. Taper off as much as you can until then. Here are ways to start to dismantle the habit:

- Stop buying cigarettes where you usually buy them. Shop elsewhere. Buy one pack at a time, not a carton.

- Switch to another brand and break brand loyalty. Expect to like this brand less.

- Go longer between cigarettes. When you smoke, put your cigarette out sooner.

- Limit cigarette breaks to one location.

- Tell at least three close friends or family members that you intend to stop. Making a declaration to others gives an incentive to succeed. They can lend emotional support. Ask them to hold you accountable for your decision. If you have smoking buddies, tell them to *never again* invite you out for a smoke. Tell them to refuse to give you cigarettes in the future, even if you ask.

Stock up on cigarette replacements – something to put in your mouth such as chewing gum, breath mints, hard candies, soda straws, cinnamon bark, or plastic coffee stirrers. Once you stop smoking, carry these at all times and use them instead of cigarettes.

Self-Hypnosis: See Yourself Smoke-Free!

Decide the exact date when you will stop smoking. When your "freedom day" arrives, smoke your last cigarette. Crumple any remaining cigarettes and throw them away. Throw away your lighters. Practice the following self-hypnosis daily for 30 days:

1. Induce trance with any method of your choosing.

2. Say the following affirmations (or something similar) as your self-suggestions:

    *   I'm glad I have stopped smoking.
    *   Smoking is behind me and my best days are ahead of me.
    *   I feel good about this achievement.
    *   All my urges and cravings for cigarettes are gone.
    *   I enjoy my freedom to be healthy.
    *   I like breathing fresh clean air into my healthy lungs!

3. Releasing imagery: Visualize a huge pile of stale, crumpled, smelly cigarettes. See a large, black-and-white signboard with a skull and crossbones on it, sticking out of the middle of this pile, above the word "POISON". See the ghosts of millions who have died from smoking rising up out of the pile of cigarettes. They are looking at you, calling out to you. "Now you are free! Celebrate and be healthy!"

    Imagine that you take a pen and small tablet out of your pocket. On each page of the tablet, write the reasons, excuses, or rationalizations you gave to perpetuate the habit. Phrase them in the past tense. Maybe you'll write, "Cigarettes helped me concentrate" or "Cigarettes helped me relax." After you write a statement on a page, rip the page off. Crumple it. Throw it into the pile of cigarettes. Each time you throw a crumpled page onto the pile, say to yourself, "Never again! Never again!"

    The ghosts vanish. On the ground beside the pile of cigarettes you see a red metal gasoline can. You pick it up. You douse the pile of cigarettes with gasoline. You light a match to it. It bursts into flame and burns brightly, releasing the odors of stale cigarettes. The papers and cigarettes disintegrate and go up in smoke. The smoke billows into the sky, taking away all urges or desires for cigarettes. The winds scatter the smoke. You walk away, free.

4. Repeat the affirmations above, in Step 2.

5. Goal imaging: Imagine living smoke-free. Make this image rich, bright, and up close. Associate into it. Realize all the advantages of smoke-free living. You enjoy the accomplishment. You are glad you stopped. You like smelling fresh and clean. No more coughing. No more hassles and expense of cigarettes. Your loved ones are happy for you. Your doctor is happy for you. Your friends compliment you. Your conscience is clear. Your senses are sharper. You have more energy. You can bound up a flight of stairs and still breathe freely and easily. You feel younger and healthier than you've felt in years!

6. Return your thoughts to the here and now. Feel enthusiasm and motivation for bringing this image into reality.

7. Access and anchor a calm state: Call forth a memory of a time when you felt totally calm and at peace (without a cigarette, of course). Associate into the memory and be there now. See what you saw. Hear what you heard. Take in the details. Let the image bring about calm, peaceful feelings within. Let your body relax completely into the calm peacefulness. Bring your thoughts into the present, staying with the calm, peaceful feelings.

8. Mental rehearsal: Imagine a location or situation where you smoked. Now, instead of smoking, you are accessing calm feelings. In the past, you smoked to feel calm in this situation, but now you find cigarettes are entirely unnecessary. The situation itself calls forth calm, peaceful feelings. Mentally rehearse your actions in this situation, feeling calm and peaceful. Affirmation: I can handle this situation without cigarettes. I'm glad to live free of a deadly habit! I feel fit and healthy!

    Repeat this step with additional locations and situations in which you previously smoked. Project your thoughts into the future, associating into each location and situation that you might encounter again – only this time, you are smoke-free. In each instance, bring about calm, peaceful feelings, and mentally rehearse what you'll say and do.[28]

9. Return your thoughts to the here and now. Reorient and open your eyes.

Preventing Relapse

The first 30 days of smoke-free living are usually the hardest. Over the next 30 days, follow these tips to make sure you remain smoke-free.

- Get adequate rest, nutrition, and exercise. Drink plenty of liquids.

- If you can, avoid stressful situations that were triggers for smoking.

- If you've smoked in your car, get your car cleaned inside and out. Let your clean, fresh-smelling car serve as a daily reminder that your body is also cleaning out all the toxins of cigarettes. Think of your body as fresh and clean, inside and out.

- You'll detect smoke smells in clothing. Wash your clothes or take them to the cleaners. You are ridding your life of all the vestiges and reminders of cigarettes.

- Alcohol is a relapse trigger. I tell my clients, "No alcohol for the first 30 days." Those who break this rule usually resume smoking.

- Keep those replacements handy and use them.

- Remind yourself that a cigarette is just a dried up, dead weed in a flimsy piece of paper. It has no power over you.

- Refuse to discuss how much you "miss" smoking or how much you "loved" it. Allow yourself one "gripe session" each day. Otherwise, drop the subject. Why? Your motivation will increase when you focus on the benefits. Be glad that you are done with the hassles, risks, and expense of cigarettes.

- See Chapter 6 on eliminating habits and addictions.

Your body is the vehicle with which you navigate your life's journey. Putting toxins into it is a sacrilege. Every smoker I've ever met regrets the day they started smoking. Every former smoker I've ever met is grateful and happy to have stopped smoking. People who smoke reduce their life expectancies by 25 years, on average. Fortunately, you can reverse much of the damage that smoking inflicts on your body. Isn't it worth it to stop smoking and live your life smoke-free?

CHAPTER 8

Achieve Your Ideal Weight

Today, there are more overweight and obese people than at any other time in history. In 2009, the U.S. Centers for Disease Control estimated the medical costs of obesity at $147 billion a year. That figure is going up as healthcare expenditure rises. The medical costs of obesity account for 9 percent of all medical spending in the U.S. Obesity is the number one reason for rising healthcare costs in most developed nations, where two-thirds of the population are overweight. Obesity is also on the rise among children and adolescents. Obesity contributes to 300,000 deaths a year in the U.S. alone. Obesity is implicated in heart disease, diabetes, high blood pressure, stroke, sleep apnea, osteoarthritis, joint problems, gall bladder disease, and some forms of cancer.

Many factors account for excessive weight gain, including genetics, hormonal imbalances, a sedentary lifestyle, and sleep disorders. All these factors make for a sluggish metabolism. Talk to your physician to learn about treatment options. Get a physical exam before attempting any weight reduction plan. Weight gain may be due to undetected illnesses that won't be addressed adequately by dietary measures or hypnosis.

In this chapter, I'll cover tips and strategies for a healthy, intelligent relationship with food. For more information on eliminating unwanted habits and starting new ones, read Chapter 6. Studies show that sleep disturbances often lead to weight gain – see Chapter 9 on how to get quality sleep. See Chapter 10 to get going on an exercise routine, so that your body burns calories more efficiently. See Chapter 11 for ways to stay motivated. If you tend to overeat because of negative thoughts about your self-worth, or because of difficult emotions, read Chapter 15 on self-esteem and Chapter 16 on emotional equanimity and resilience.

Get Smart about HGI Foods

When it comes to weight management, it's not only the number of calories you consume that matters; it's the *type* of calories you consume. One of the main causes of weight gain is poor nutrition – eating too much of the wrong *kinds* of food. Sugars, fats, starches, many processed foods, and alcohol break down rapidly in the digestive system, converting to sugar. Sugar has little nutritional value. Sugars carry a high glycemic index (HGI). HGI foods are stored as fat because the body gets energy more efficiently from proteins and high fiber foods that digest slowly.[29] A steady intake of HGI foods puts the body on the sugar roller-coaster.

Here's a highly simplified explanation. The body converts HGI calories to simple sugars in the digestive tract. As sugars flood the bloodstream, the pancreas pumps out insulin to bring down sugar levels. Suppose this happens several times daily. The pancreas goes into overdrive, putting out more insulin. Sugar levels drop too low, too fast. The result is fatigue and difficulty concentrating. Many overweight people interpret fatigue as a need for more sugar. They keep riding the roller-coaster of sugar highs and sugar lows.

When the cycle becomes chronic, the resulting condition is hypoglycemia. Over time, however, the pancreas can no longer sustain the heightened activity. It wears out and stops producing insulin. The resulting condition is type 2 diabetes. Sugar overload holds other dangers as well. It impairs immunity and disrupts the production of hormones, creating an acidic internal environment. The body tries to compensate by increasing alkalinity. It does so by removing calcium and other minerals from the bones. Sugar also causes elevated levels of cholesterol and triglycerides, increasing the risk for heart disease.[30]

Sugar is addictive because it briefly elevates serotonin: a neurotransmitter that produces positive feelings. If you decide to eliminate sugars from your diet, you may experience a few days of sugar withdrawal. Eat fresh fruits and vegetables for about two weeks and your internal chemistry levels will adapt and become more stable. Unfortunately, the typical diet in most developed nations is abundant with HGI foods. To attain a healthy weight, start replacing HGI foods with high-fiber foods and low-fat proteins. Table 2 shows the types of foods in each category.

Table 2 is not a dietary recommendation. Your nutrition plan should meet your individual needs. If you aren't sure how to obtain healthy, balanced nutrition, consult a nutritionist. The purpose of this table is to show the HGI foods most likely to cause blood sugar problems and weight gain, as opposed to foods that break down more slowly in the digestive tract.

If I could give one recommendation for a healthy weight, it would be this: eat HGI foods sparingly. It's my observation that overweight people eat far too many HGI foods. High-fiber foods and proteins, on the other hand, take longer to break down in the digestive tract. With these types of food, you can enjoy feeling hungry less often and maintain energy throughout the day.

Table 2 HGI Foods versus Sources of Fiber and Low-Fat Proteins

High Glycemic Index Foods	**Sources of Fiber and Low-Fat Proteins**
• Potatoes and white rice • Baked goods made of sugar and refined white flour: cookies, cakes, pies, and pastries • Candies • Ice cream, sherbets, frozen yoghurts • Pasta, pizza, and breads • Crackers, chips, and crisps • Many processed foods • Sugary cereals • Colas, energy drinks, and fruit drinks • Alcoholic drinks • Sugar-based additives, including high fructose corn syrup, barley malt, galactose, agave nectar, honey, maple syrup, corn sweetener, dextrine, rice syrup, glucose, sucrose, and dextrose	• Most fresh fruits, dried fruits, or fruits packed in their own juices • Fresh vegetables, raw or steamed • Beans and legumes • Nuts • Whole grains • Lean meats, fowl, and fish • Low-fat dairy products

Tips for Sensible Eating

Here are my best tips for sensible eating – and none of them call for dieting! They tell you how to reprogram eating patterns for an intelligent relationship with food.[31]

- **Cup your hands together and look at them.** The space between your cupped hands should be about the size of a large grapefruit. This gives a visual idea of what a full stomach can comfortably hold. Eat only what your stomach can comfortably accommodate.

- **Eat less in restaurants.** Most restaurants serve over-large portions. If the food is delicious, and you've paid for it, it's tempting to eat it all, and waddle out, feeling stuffed. Instead, ask for a take-home box, and place half the meal in it to have later. Alternatively, you can split your meal with another person at your table. You can order soup and salad, instead of a whole meal. Ask the wait staff to hold the complimentary breads.

- **Drink water before you eat.** You'll feel less hungry. Your stomach will fill up faster. This way, you can eat less and still feel full.

- **Manage portions.** Choose smaller portions. Leave space on your plate or eat from a salad plate instead of a dinner plate. If you load your plate up with more than you can eat, it's okay to leave food on your plate. Although I don't advise anyone to waste food, it's better to throw it out or save it for another meal than to consume calories you don't need.

- **Devote your full attention to eating.** Of course it's not possible to always do this. Nevertheless, if you eat while driving, watching television, or reading, you aren't giving full attention to the food or to the feeling of food in your body. Such habits lead to overeating and ignoring physical signals of fullness.

- **Eat slowly.** It takes 15 to 20 minutes for the stomach to send a message to the brain that it's time to stop eating. If you eat slowly, your brain can catch up with your stomach. You can feel full before you've overstuffed. Take small bites, chew thoroughly and concentrate on the taste and texture of the food. Pause between bites, putting your fork down, taking a deep breath, having a drink of water, and conversing with dinner companions.

- **Rethink the meaning of overeating.** When you overeat, do you use that experience as feedback or do you berate yourself? When you overeat, notice the physical discomfort. Instead of berating yourself, make a decision to remember those feelings. Let them serve as feedback to eat moderately in the future.

- **Ask yourself, "If I didn't spend so much time obsessing about food and weight, what would I be doing instead?"** Sometimes we invest in negative habits because we are in denial about the fact that we could discover our true potentials and experience the joy of pursuing the purposes that would make our lives meaningful and fulfilling.

Self-Hypnosis: Sensible Eating

This self-hypnosis session incorporates many of the ideas above. Here are the steps:

1. Sit or recline comfortably. Induce trance with any method of your choosing.

2. In your visual field, see two squares side by side. In the left square, place images of HGI foods. The square might resemble a collage. Include your most problematic foods. In the right square, place images of high-fiber and low-fat protein foods. This square could also resemble a collage. Alter the submodalities of the images. Focus on the left square. Make the images dull and dim. Move the square back, further away. Focus on the right square. Move it in close so that you really see the colors and textures of the foods. See that they are fresh, flavorful, and nutritious. Let your unconscious program your body so that you prefer these slenderizing foods. Let your visual field go blank.

3. Affirmation: I enjoy slenderizing foods!

4. Goal imaging: See an image of your future self at your ideal weight. Make this image rich, clear, and focused. Step into this image, feeling

healthy and confident, knowing it was worth the effort to look and feel this good. Imagine the differences in your life. Visualize walking into a clothing store and selecting a new dress, pair of pants, or suit in your favorite size. Imagine stepping onto the scale in your doctor's exam room, and seeing the numbers register just where you like to see them. Imagine standing in front of a full length mirror and feeling satisfied with the changes you see. You are amazed! Visualize a social gathering where friends compliment you on your healthier appearance. You feel happy! Imagine walking onto the dance floor with your sweetheart, feeling attractive and confident. You feel glad about all the ways you have changed your habits to achieve your ideal weight.

5. Affirmation: I feel delighted to be maintaining my ideal weight and my favorite body size!

6. Look backwards in time, from the future, to the present. See what you did to reach your favorite size. You discovered how to say "NO!" to fattening, sugary, starchy foods. You changed your food preferences to nutritious, slenderizing foods. You downsized your portions. You put care into shopping and meal planning. You've made it a habit to get quality sleep and adequate exercise. You watched the extra pounds melt away one by one, week after week. You followed your plan consistently. Even when you made mistakes or got sidetracked, you renewed your intention and commitment.

7. Return your thoughts to the here and now. Reorient and open your eyes.

Self-Hypnosis: The NLP Slender Eating Strategy

The NLP Slender Eating Strategy was developed by NLP trainer Connirae Andreas.[32] It helps you to eat according to your body's natural signals, instead of in response to external stimuli. You can apply this strategy each time you think about eating. Here you can practice it in self-hypnosis as a mental rehearsal:

1. Induce trance with any method of your choosing.

2. Imagine you are thinking about food. Decide if you really feel hungry or if you are thinking about food because of an external trigger or an

emotion. If you aren't really hungry, do something else instead. If you *are* hungry, go to Step 3.

3. Decide what to eat. Concentrate on the sensations in your mouth. What would taste good? Put your hand on your stomach. What would feel good in your stomach? What is your body telling you it would like to eat? It's okay to limit your selections to what you have on hand in the kitchen or what's on the menu in a restaurant.

4. Think ahead. Imagine eating the food you selected. How will it feel and taste in your mouth? How will it feel in your stomach? How will you feel an hour after you've eaten that food? Will it be satisfying? If so, go on to Step 5. If not, test out other options until you find one that is acceptable.

5. Imagine you've now decided *what* to eat. Next, decide *how much* to eat. Place your hand on your stomach. How much of this food will give you a satisfied feeling of fullness in your stomach? You'll get an intuitive indication of just the right amount of food to satisfy your hunger.

6. Imagine that you start eating slowly and mindfully. Take small bites, concentrating on each one. Really taste the food and feel the texture. Pause between bites. Chew your food thoroughly. Be aware of chewing, tasting, and swallowing. Between bites, put down your fork and breathe deeply. Place your hand on your stomach and feel the sensations of fullness gathering there. You will automatically stop when you feel satisfied. When you eat mindfully, you enjoy the food more, so you eat less.

7. Imagine that you stop eating when you feel full. It doesn't matter if others are still eating, or if there's additional food on the table or on your plate. It doesn't matter if someone encourages you to eat more or have a second helping. Just say "No, thanks." Get up and leave the table if necessary. You could sip water while others finish. At a restaurant, ask the wait staff to remove your plate. You are learning to eat according to your body's innate communication patterns.

8. Return your thoughts to the here and now. Reorient and open your eyes.

Change Your Thoughts about Food

A few final thoughts about food. In my opinion, we are far too cavalier about food. We treat it as a commodity instead of a blessing. By eating mindfully, you can take time to appreciate each meal as a sensual experience. Smell the fragrances and aromas of food. Look at the colors. The most nutritious meals have a variety of colors. As you eat, concentrate on the flavor and texture of the food in your mouth. Enjoy the feelings as your appetite is satisfied and your stomach begins to fill.

Food is essential to life. Eating can be a sacred act. When you sit down at a table, consider, for a moment, the time and effort that went into the meal before you. Bless those whose labor made it possible for this food to arrive at your table. Have gratitude that you and your family can afford this food. Feel thankful for the care that went into the planning and preparation of this meal. If you are eating meat, have reverence for the animal that was once a living, breathing, sentient being whose life was sacrificed for your enjoyment and sustenance. To have food on the table is an amazing measure of abundance not enjoyed by all in the world. Honor the food you eat. Honor the body you nourish.

CHAPTER 9

Quality Sleep

Quality sleep is essential for health, vitality, and performance. Without it, motivation and self-confidence ebb, energy drops, and performance suffers. In our often sleep-deprived society, many people underestimate the value of regular and adequate sleep. In fact, some think their ability to get by on little sleep is an indication of their work ethic (they work such long hours) or social popularity (they party 'til the wee hours of the morning). Not so. Most people can sacrifice sleep occasionally, but to do so on a regular basis spells trouble.

According to the U.S. National Institutes of Health, 70 million Americans have insomnia, sometimes transient, sometimes chronic. Women have it more frequently than men. In fact, the U.S Centers for Disease Control have declared insufficient sleep a public health epidemic. The National Sleep Foundation estimates the direct costs of insomnia at nearly $14 billion annually. Those costs include treatment, healthcare, hospitalization, and nursing home care. Indirect costs such as lost productivity and property damage from accidents come close to $28 billion annually.

How important is sleep? Studies by the National Center on Sleep Disorders Research have shown that sleep deprivation leads to confusion, reduced reasoning, and diminished coping skills. Long periods of inadequate sleep contribute to lowered immunity, cardiovascular disease, excess weight, hormonal imbalances, reduced concentration, poor memory, cognitive impairment, and poor coordination.[33] Drowsiness is a major cause of automobile accidents. Obviously, sufficient sleep is necessary for safety, productivity, and problem-solving as well as health, healing, and tissue repair.

Insomnia can be caused by stress, tension, and poor habits, or medical problems such as allergies, acid reflux, pain, depression, or anxiety. If your sleep problems persist, see a physician. For severe sleep problems, your physician might refer you to a sleep specialist or a sleep study clinic.

Before choosing any over-the-counter sleep aid, consult your doctor first about possible interactions with supplements and prescription medications. If stress from psychological trauma, unhappy relationships, anger, guilt, or frustration keep you up at night, consult a psychotherapist.

Tips for A Good Night's Sleep

In April 2009, in the wake of the international economic crisis that began the previous year, the *Los Angeles Times* reported a surprising statistic. In 2008, in the U.S. alone, prescriptions for sleep medications topped 56 million, an increase of 54 percent from 2004.[34] That statistic doesn't even take into account over-the-counter sleep medications! It seems surprising that so many people need prescriptions and over-the-counter drugs to bring about the body's natural response of sleep. Yet somehow, for large numbers of people, the pressures of daily life have robbed them of the ability to fall asleep without a pill – and sleep medications can cause side-effects such as memory loss, dependency, and next-day drowsiness. Something is wrong with this picture.

There is no doubt that stress is a major contributor to sleep disturbances. However, it is possible to recover the ability to sleep without medication. The tips that follow will tell you how.[35]

- **Avoid nicotine, alcohol, and caffeine in the late evening.** Nicotine and caffeine are stimulants that keep most people awake. Alcohol may seem relaxing, but many people fall asleep after one or two drinks only to waken two or three hours later, unable to return to sleep. Alcohol interferes with sleep because even in small amounts it dehydrates the brain, making sleep impossible.

- **Drink water.** Dehydration can play havoc with sleep patterns, so drink sufficient water during the day and before going to bed.

- **Keep regular hours.** An erratic or irregular schedule of getting up and going to bed will throw off the body's natural biological clock that governs the cycle of waking and sleeping. It's best to maintain regular, predictable hours for getting up and going to bed, even on weekends and vacations.

- **Make your bedroom conducive to sleep and rest.** The ideal sleep environment is a quiet, tranquil place of soft colors, simplicity and order. Your mattress should be comfortable. Adequate air circulation and humidity are a benefit. The room should be dark because darkness facilitates the brain's sleeping functions. If you sleep during the day, or if your home is in a well-lit area, put shades and curtains on the windows. Perhaps you'd like to wear a sleep-mask or eye pillow as well.

- **Make your bedroom as quiet as possible.** Some people enjoy listening to soft music or recordings of rhythmic sounds, such as rain drops, to increase drowsiness. If your home is in a noisy area, such as a city street, consider investing in triple-pane insulated windows. Perhaps a white-noise machine will help. You can achieve the same effect by tuning a radio to an open channel with only static. If your bed partner snores, you might want to discuss alternative sleeping arrangements.

- **Maintain a bedtime routine that allows you to wind down the day.** Your routine might include walking the dog, checking the stove, locking doors, turning off lights, setting the alarm, brushing your teeth, and so on. Such simple tasks give peace of mind and a feeling that the day is complete.

- **Before bedtime, transition to pleasant, quiet, restful activities.** Avoid bedtime snacking, strenuous physical activity before bedtime, playing computer games, or watching television until bedtime. All of these stimulate the brain and are not conducive to sleep. Instead, use the 30 minutes or so before bedtime to stretch, do some deep breathing exercises, listen to soft music, meditate, pray, write in a journal, read a novel or poetry, or indulge in a hot bath or shower.

- **Don't fret about sleep problems.** If you worry about not sleeping, the tension that accompanies worry may be *causing* sleeplessness – thus creating a self-fulfilling prophecy. To "work" at getting to sleep will prove an exercise in futility. Bedtime is not the time for problem-solving or dwelling on frustrations. The less you think about, the better. Sleep should be a time of soothing comfort and effortless relaxation. Occupy your mind with pleasant thoughts.

- **Consider natural aids to sleep.** Melatonin helps some people to regulate their sleep cycles. The usual dosage is 75 milligrams, taken orally at bedtime. Do not take melatonin with supplements containing magnesium or zinc because this may produce an adverse reaction. Many people rely on a glass of milk before bedtime. The vitamin D in milk activates the brain's own sedative, tryptophan. Chamomile tea is also relaxing.

- **Keep a small notepad beside the bed.** If a worrisome thought occurs, or if you suddenly think of something you should remember for the next day, write it down. Then put the thought out of your mind, knowing you'll handle the matter tomorrow.

- **Consider aromatherapy.** Essential oils of geranium, lavender, marjoram, sandalwood, and patchouli facilitate rest and relaxation. You can obtain these oils as a spray mist for your pillow or in powder form as an additive to a warm bath, just before bed. If you burn aromatherapy candles or heat essential oils in a candle diffuser, use care. Make sure the flame is out before you go to sleep.

Self-Hypnosis: Restful, Restorative Sleep

Induction Method 6 (Progressive Relaxation), in Chapter 5, is an excellent relaxation method for falling asleep. With hypnosis, I teach my clients how to combine relaxation methods with positive self-suggestions, to fall asleep easily and effortlessly. Here are the steps:

1. Begin by getting comfortable. Close your eyes. Take in a long, slow, deep breath and slowly exhale. Take in a second long, slow, deep breath and slowly exhale again. Take in a third long, slow, deep breath and slowly exhale.

2. Put aside the cares and concerns of the day. Visualize a large box in which you can dump any worries, unresolved issues, or unfinished business. Put whatever you want into the box, seal it, and push it under the bed or into the closet.

3. Go into trance with progressive relaxation (see Chapter 5).

4. Say the following self-suggestions:
    - I fall asleep easily and effortlessly whenever I want to fall asleep.
    - I sleep well throughout the night.
    - I enjoy a restorative, rejuvenating sleep.
    - I wake up when I want to wake up.
    - I wake in the morning feeling alert and refreshed.

5. Deepen your relaxation by counting from one to five, saying each number on the outward breath. Relax more deeply with each number.

6. Deepen your relaxation again using the staircase induction in Chapter 5.

7. Repeat the self-suggestions in Step 4.

8. Deepen your relaxation by counting from one to ten, saying each number on the outward breath. Relax more deeply with each number.

9. Let your arms and legs feel heavy and motionless. Imagine floating on a soft, fluffy, white cloud across a blue sky. You drift through a silent landscape of sky and clouds. You feel peaceful and calm. Repeat the self-suggestions in Step 4.

10. Repeat Steps 3 through 8 until you fall asleep.

Adequate Sleep Offers Many Advantages

A good night's sleep renews the mind and body. Your thinking is sharper when you feel well rested. During sleep, your unconscious solves problems and processes information. During sleep, your body makes repairs. During sleep, the body releases hormones necessary to healthy metabolism.

Surely you've heard about someone who decided to "sleep on a problem" and woke up the next day with the solution? Creative artists and scientists often report that their best ideas have come to them during a dream or upon awakening. While sleep requirements vary according to age and health, most people require seven to eight hours of sleep each night to function at their best. Are you getting your nightly requirement?

CHAPTER 10

Start Exercising!

If all the benefits of exercise could be squeezed into a pill, it would be a miracle drug – the "rejuvenation pill." Everyone would want it. People would pay thousands of dollars for the extraordinary advantages, which come with no side-effects! No one would want to be without it! So why don't more people get off their behinds and exercise?

Newspapers, books, television shows, and magazines extol the benefits of physical activity as a means to fitness and a longer life. In every town and city in the U.S. you can find bike paths, jogging trails, health clubs, gyms, racquet clubs, tennis courts, aerobics classes, dance studios, martial arts classes, and community recreation facilities. You would surmise that the country is caught up in a frenzy of fitness.

Although people increasingly understand the value of exercise, it's also true that obesity has reached epidemic proportions in many developed countries. Life doesn't have to be that way for *you*. You don't have to be a couch potato!

The Benefits of Exercise[36]

Regular exercise brings more than a better physique. Exercise can help you sleep better, manage stress more effectively, strengthen your heart, prevent osteoporosis, burn calories, decrease your appetite, improve your skin, and bolster your self-esteem. Physical activity, combined with good nutrition, can actually slow the aging process itself.

Let's look more closely at the rewards of exercise. The physical benefits of exercise are:

- **Improved circulation, a stronger heart, and stronger lung capacity:** Aerobic activity works the heart muscles, increases blood flow, and makes the lungs pump harder – strengthening the entire cardiovascular system.

- **Healthier skin:** Exercise increases circulation, bringing blood to the surface, delivering nutrients and flushing away toxins. Skin gets a youthful glow!

- **Neurogenesis:** Recent studies show that exercise helps grow new brain cells and increases brain proteins in mice. Research is underway to find similar results in humans.[37]

- **Prevention of osteoporosis:** Weight-bearing exercise, such as walking, strengthens bones and can slow loss of bone density due to aging.

- **Increased metabolism:** Exercise burns calories and keeps the metabolic rate high for hours, even after the activity has ended.

- **Increased muscle tone:** If you are dieting without exercising, you're losing muscle instead of fat. To retain muscle, you must exercise. Muscle tissue is denser than fat and takes up less space, so you look slimmer, with more muscle and less fat.

- **Rehabilitation from muscular-skeletal injuries:** Under the supervision of a sports physician or physical therapist, targeted exercises and movement can facilitate repair of damaged muscles, ligaments, and tendons. Sometimes even old injuries can improve with proper exercise.

Exercise also gives you these psychological benefits:

- **Relief from stress and mild, transitory depression:** Exercise is a healthy way to work off frustration. It gives "time out" from the demands of work and family. Increased circulation pumps oxygen to the brain for clearer thinking. Whole body activity stimulates both hemispheres of the brain, which can have a calming effect.

- **Increased self-esteem:** Meeting a physical challenge – like finishing a 10-kilometer race or hiking a mountain trail – brings the exhilaration of accomplishment and an enhanced sense of competence and mastery. Some people enjoy the camaraderie of team sports and the shared fun of group activity. Some enjoy the improved grace that comes from activities involving precision movement such as dance, swimming, or gymnastics.

There is no pill, no medical treatment, and no cosmetic preparation that can equal the benefits of regular physical exercise. Given these fantastic benefits, you can't pass it up! Exercise is absolutely essential to your health and well-being. So why don't *you* get off your behind and exercise?

Tips for Starting an Exercise Routine

If you are not yet into an exercise routine, here are some ways to get started on a sensible regimen that will transform mind, body, and spirit. The key to success is to set reasonable, incremental goals and to build strength and stamina slowly and safely over time. Follow these guidelines to developing an exercise routine:

- **Consult with your physician first:** Get a complete physical exam and ask your physician about the types of exercise that are safe for you.

- **Choose a mix of activities:** Ideally, you want an exercise routine that includes stretching exercises for flexibility, aerobic activity for cardiovascular fitness, and resistance exercises for strength and toning.

- **Hire a trainer:** Consult with a personal trainer who can design an exercise routine based on your age, physical condition, and fitness goals. A trainer is especially important if you plan to use weights or exercise machines. She can help you start out at the proper speed and level of resistance, show you the proper postures and movements, and teach you how to avoid injury.

- **Get the right gear:** Make sure to wear proper clothing for your activity. If you use equipment, it should be in excellent condition and well maintained.

- **Warm up and stretch:** To start your routine, spend about 5 minutes warming up – for example, walking in place or freestyle dancing – to get the blood circulating to muscles and to loosen up joints. Then stretch slowly until you feel some resistance and hold each stretch for a count of 10 to 20 seconds. Warming up helps avoid muscle sprains.

- **Start slowly and pay attention to your body's responses:** During the first days and weeks of a new exercise routine, be careful and don't push too hard. Limit initial workouts to a few minutes of light activity. If you feel fatigue or pain, stop, rest, and resume tomorrow. Build strength and stamina over several weeks or months. Increase the demands on your body gradually.

- **Make it fun:** Do exercise you enjoy. Exercise alone in the privacy of your home or with a friend. Go to a gym or join a class. If your routine gets dull, build in variety. Exercise to music, walk with your pooch, bicycle with your child, or take dance lessons with your sweetheart.

- **Chart your progress:** Put a chart on your refrigerator that shows how many sit-ups you do each day, how many miles you walk, or how many minutes you spend on the treadmill. Or just put a big gold star on the calendar for every day you exercise. Soon you will like what you see!

- **Integrate movement into your daily routine:** You'll get more from exercise (and burn additional calories) if you stay active during the day. If you sit for most of the day, take breaks at least every hour to stand up, stretch, take a few deep breaths, and walk around.

- **Make an appointment with yourself:** Schedule exercise time on your daily calendar and give that time top priority. Keep the engagement, as if it were an appointment to receive a million dollars, meet with world leaders, interview for your dream job, or go on a date with someone you adore. Get into a daily routine so you actually begin to look forward to exercising. Don't miss it for anything except an emergency. Don't let others talk you out of it. Make exercise time sacred and non-negotiable. Exercise is for you, to make you feel good and look good!

- **Set a milestone:** You can increase your motivation by setting physical milestones for yourself that will require you to work out regularly so that you can meet each one. It helps if your milestone involves a public display of your strength and fortitude. This way, you are "in training" for it. When I was jogging, for example, I signed up for 10K races – usually one each month. I paid for each one, cleared my calendar for it, and even invited a few friends to jog with me, to make sure I had a strong commitment. As each race loomed before me, I felt motivated to keep up my routine so that I could finish the race with a decent time. Your goal might be to have the strength to spend a day at Disney World with your grandchildren, to walk in a fundraising drive, or to dance in a musical. Just make sure the actual date is close enough that you can feel the pressure to be in shape for it.

- **Join a class:** Some people like the social atmosphere of a class and the fact that it takes place on a schedule. Sometimes it's easier to get there when you've paid for it, too.

- **Find a buddy:** Find a buddy to exercise with and make a commitment to each other. I know two women who walk together every morning, three times a week. I know three men who golf together on Friday afternoons. Knowing that someone else is counting on you is a powerful motivator.

- **Join a team:** A team is a group of buddies, all counting on each other, encouraging each other, and expecting each other to show up and give their best. For some, teamwork offers an irresistible incentive. If you like team camaraderie and competition with other teams, then your sport might be soccer, baseball, crew, or basketball.

Self-Hypnosis: Get Motivated with the NLP New Behavior Generator

Self-motivation is a complex process of (1) recognizing sufficiently compelling incentives, (2) establishing a belief that certain actions will cause those incentives to materialize, (3) planning how to take those actions, and (4) engaging in those actions sufficiently to accomplish results. Motivation requires strategies for consistently accessing resourceful states that compel action.

The New Behavior Generator, developed by John Grinder, is an NLP process for choosing a new behavior and motivating yourself to carry it out. The adaptation below draws from many NLP sources.[38] Before you begin, develop a reasonable exercise plan, following the tips above. Here are the steps:

1. Induce and deepen trance with any method of your choosing.

2. Give yourself incentives to exercise. Visualize the rewards or satis-factions you expect to get from exercise. You might choose stamina, vitality, attractiveness, feeling younger, a flat stomach, or feeling confident wearing a swimsuit.

3. Goal imaging: Visualize your incentives fulfilled. Associate into each image. Imagine exactly how you would look and feel. What would you be doing differently? Make these images moving, vivid, and realis-tic. Keep enhancing each scenario, making it more vivid (with sights, sounds, and feelings) until you get a "Wow!" feeling!

4. Access a resourceful state of passion. What is an activity that you pursue passionately? You know: something that excites you just to think about it. Access a memory of that activity. Be there. Feel your passion for it! Notice how you look forward to that activity. What do you say to yourself? What kinds of images do you make in your mind? You are accessing a state of passion. Anchor it with the word, "PASSION!" Give yourself the suggestion that when you say the word "PASSION" to yourself, you'll return to this state.

5. Access a strategy for self-discipline. What is an activity that you pur-sue routinely, with a firm, steady, self-discipline? You know: some-thing that you may not always like, but the rewards are such that you do it consistently and willingly. Remember a recent time when you managed yourself into doing it. Be there now. Study how you got yourself to do it. What was your strategy? In other words, what exactly did you tell yourself? What did you say that moved you to act? What internal tone of voice did you use? How did you arrange to do it? How did you keep yourself on task? What images did you make in your mind? Note all the essential elements of your strategy for SELF-DISCIPLINE.

6. Mental rehearsal: Visualize a movie of yourself exercising. Imagine you are the director of the movie. Watch yourself go through the movements, flexing and contracting your muscles, breathing, and

concentrating. Keep modifying the movie until it looks realistic, doable, and appealing.

7. Step into the movie. What do you see? What do you hear? Imagine the movement, the breathing, the concentration, and other details.

8. Step out of the movie and evaluate it. What can you change to make it more appealing? Step into the movie again. Replay it with any improvements.

9. Step out of the movie. Watch the movie again, this time feeling PASSION! Step into the movie. Be there, exercising with PASSION! Notice how PASSION changes the quality of the experience!

10. Mental rehearsal: Step out of the movie. Imagine future scenarios in which you are exercising consistently with PASSION!

11. Affirmation: I exercise with PASSION!

12. Pick the day and time for the next time you plan to exercise. Imagine that as the time draws near, you feel increasing PASSION for it. You are looking forward to it with PASSION. When you think about that exercise appointment with yourself, apply the elements of your strategy for SELF-DISCIPLINE. How will you manage your thinking so that you actually keep that appointment? What do you think about? What do you say to yourself? What images do you visualize?

13. Mental rehearsal: Visualize that you are exercising. Be there now. See the environment. Hear the sounds. Imagine the movement – the muscles flexing and contracting. Imagine your breathing and heartbeat. You might be sweating or groaning, cheering yourself on, or coaching yourself. As you exercise, keep reminding yourself that you are now creating the rewards and satisfactions that you visualized in Step 3. Keep flashing on those same goal images that provide compelling incentives. Keep getting back to that "Wow!" feeling.

14. Your exercise session is over. You feel flushed with exertion and happy with the accomplishment. Realize that you could really *miss* having this feeling. Look forward to the next exercise session, knowing you'll apply your SELF-DISCIPLINE strategy again and maintain your PASSION!

15. Return to the present. Multiply this scenario into the future, antici-
    pating many sequential exercise sessions. Here's how. Take the sce-
    nario from Step 12. Imagine holding it in your hand as a DVD. Multiply
    the DVD many times over so that you have a huge stack of nearly
    identical DVDs – all movies of you exercising with PASSION. Toss the
    DVDs out into your future so that the scenario you just visualized
    is now replicated many times. See future instances in which you are
    exercising, applying SELF-DISCIPLINE, feeling PASSION, and com-
    ing closer and closer to those satisfying benefits and rewards. Wow!

16. Return your thoughts to the present. Reorient and open your eyes.

Obviously, travel, emergencies, and illness will occasionally throw you
off your routine. Take it in stride. That's what professional athletes do.
As soon as you can, get back to your routine. For more ideas and self-
hypnosis strategies for motivation, see the next chapter.

Consider Additional Options for Exercise as You Age

Even if you enjoy a particular sport or exercise tremendously, it's not
always possible to continue it all your life. Because of changes in your
schedule, responsibilities, or health, you may need to change the type of
exercise you do from year to year.

I was a jogger for years and loved it. Then in my forties I had a minor back
injury and later, arthritis in a knee, making any impactful exercise very
painful. It took a while to find other forms of exercise that I really liked.
Today, I work out at a neighborhood gym, cycling on a reclining bike
and lifting weights. If your favorite sport is no longer an option, don't
give up. Adapt and find another to enjoy. Fortunately, there are forms
of safe exercise for people of any age and even for those with physical
impairment.

CHAPTER 11

Maximize Your Motivation!

Motivation is essential to personal mastery and self-actualization. When people don't do what they say they want to do, it means they don't know how to consistently motivate themselves to take action toward their goals. In this chapter, we'll first briefly explore the psychology of motivation. Then I will tell you how to view failure as a stepping stone toward success. I'll give you my favorite self-motivation tips. Then I'll provide self-hypnosis methods for maximizing your motivation. With these methods you'll:

- Visualize a conversation with your future self.

- Imagine a day in which you are faithfully engaged in your desired outcome.

- Identify with a role model.

To begin this chapter, choose a project or a behavior for which you want maximum motivation. Outline a plan of action steps. Then apply the self-hypnosis methods in this chapter for motivation to accomplish your goal.

Tips to Maximize Motivation

I've always been intrigued about the magic of motivation. I've read about it, written about it, and when I incorporated my practice, I named it Motivational Strategies®. Among all the tips for motivation I've collected, here are my favorites.

- **Assess your readiness.** In Chapter 6, I wrote about Prochaska's Transtheoretical Model of Change, which shows the six stages of readiness for behavioral change. Review these steps and determine your own stage and what you can do to move to the next.

- **Begin with the end in mind.** In *The Seven Habits of Highly Effective People*, Stephen Covey told his readers that the first habit of effective living is to "Begin with the end in mind."[39] Many motivational authors and speakers have echoed this excellent advice. On a day-to-day basis, as you work toward an outcome, you may not always see an immediate result. Maintain your vision of the goal and link it to your values. Values are inherently motivating because they are the ideals for which we strive. To identify values, we can ask ourselves questions about meaning, what matters, and what's worthwhile and important.

- **Take small steps.** Take small steps in the direction of your outcomes. In *One Small Step Can Change Your Life*, author, business consultant, and behavioral health instructor, Robert Maurer, advised his readers that small steps lead to big results.[40] His simple tenet is that we accomplish large projects by starting with small, doable, steps, and by making steady progress and continuous improvement.

  Small steps are easier to accommodate and less overwhelming than giant leaps. Small steps allow us to experience initial successes that whet the appetite for additional progress. Small steps keep us from making huge mistakes or over-committing. They provide feedback for determining the next decision or action.

- **Give yourself credit for progress.** Sometimes, a new client will say, "I want to accomplish my goals, but I just have no motivation." I say, "Well, you came here today. You had the motivation to make an appointment and show up! That's a start!" To *stay* motivated, give yourself credit for progress, no matter how small.

- **Ask quality questions.** The answers you get depend on the questions you ask. In *QBQ: The Question Behind the Question*, John Miller, a leading expert on organizational development, wrote that when things go wrong, most of us resort to blaming, complaining, and procrastinating.[41] We perpetuate problems by asking "lousy questions," such as "Why does this happen?" or "Who's at fault?" or "When will this problem go away?" Such questions lead to "victim thinking."

Quality questions, on the other hand, begin with "What" or "How." They contain an "I" and focus on constructive action. Examples are: "What can I do?" and "What can I contribute?" and "How can I adapt?" Quality questions offer choice and point thinking toward solutions. Quality questions help us to focus on the one person we can change – our self.

- **Develop habits.** Whatever you want to do, it becomes easier when you make it a habit. You must do something consistently and daily for at least three or four weeks before it begins to feel like a habit. In *Falling Awake*, educator and coach, Dave Ellis, gave his readers three steps to forming a habit: commitment, monitoring, and practice.[42]

  - *Commitment:* Your commitment must be authentic, intense, and linked to your values. Do you really want your outcome? Is this a good time to make this change? Are you doing it of your own initiative? If you can say yes to these questions, then your commitment is authentic.

  - *Monitoring:* Monitoring progress makes your efforts more real and visible. Post a chart where you will look at it daily. It is a visible reminder of your progress. Choose whatever measure gives a clear indication of your efforts, so that you can see lapses and correct them, as well as celebrate milestones.

  - *Practice:* Practice means that you persist, despite setbacks. If you get off track, observe your behavior without reproach and recommit. Each day is a new day to begin creating the habits that support your goals.

- **To thine own self be true.** Don't start a plan just because someone else wants you to. Do it because *you* want to. When you formulate your plan, adapt it to your personality, needs, and schedule. Do things in your own way and work at your own pace, so that you are less likely to sabotage your efforts.

Transform Failure into Feedback

The possibility of failure can constitute a formidable obstacle to progress in any significant endeavor. Sometimes we hesitate to move forward with a plan because we fear failure. Maybe we failed before and hate the thought of starting over again and making the same mistakes. The fear of failure can lead to discouragement and giving up.

Failure can stop you in your tracks, *unless* you have a strategy to keep going. In *The NLP Coach*, coaching consultants and NLP practitioners Ian McDermott and Wendy Jago wrote that failure, like success, has a structure.[43] Both leave a trail of clues as to what went right and what went wrong. People who accomplish their goals have a distinct response to failure: they examine it with curiosity to retrieve useful information for modifying their plans and making different choices. They define failure as an unexpected detour in the journey toward the goal. The detour may make the journey longer and more arduous, but eventually they get back on track and keep going.

Conversely, others regard failure as a reason to quit. They may perceive failure as an indication of personal inadequacy, inability, or incompetence. Worse, some people keep repeating the behaviors that led to failure in the first place, each time hoping for (but not getting) a different result. A crucial element in success is to regard "failure" (lack of success) as a source of feedback. "Failure is a form of feedback," is a basic presupposition of NLP. Instead of giving up, get *curious* about failure. Regard it as an opportunity to acquire more information about how to succeed. Ask questions such as: "How did I get this result? Where did the mistakes occur? What was I thinking that led to that choice? What did I not know?"

When you analyze a failure with these questions, get specific with your answers. Don't say, "I just messed up." Don't generalize, as in, "Well, I can't do anything right." Answer the questions with an eye for the crucial details that made the *difference* between success and failure. Try out various scenarios: "If this one element had been different, would the result have been the same?" With specific information, you can reconstruct the chain of events to identify corrective action. Learn from the information and apply it.

Self-Hypnosis: A Conversation with Your "Future Self"

A compelling future is a visualization of a future that is so attractive, so vivid, so essentially tied to personal values that it is absolutely irresistible. With a compelling future, people persevere, strive, and endure hardships. A compelling future evokes an emotional attachment that magnetizes attention and energies. One way to make the future seem compelling is to envision a future self who has accomplished the goal. She can give you advice and encouragement. In this self-hypnosis session, you can preview your future through the eyes of this future self (a wisdom figure). Here are the steps:

1. Induce and deepen trance with any method of your choice.

2. Imagine you are clairvoyantly looking into your future. Your future self materializes. She is the "you" who has achieved your outcome. This other "you" has exerted consistent action and accomplished the goal, showing you the unmistakable evidence. This other "you" is your friend, mentor, and coach, here to share what she has learned.

3. Speak to this other "you." Ask questions such as:

    *   How did you do it? What steps did you take?
    *   What is it like to have accomplished this goal?
    *   How can I improve on my plan?
    *   What have you learned that I don't yet know?
    *   How can I move through discouragement and setbacks?
    *   What is the main problem I need to solve, and how shall I do it?
    *   What additional advice do you want to give me at this point?

    Quiet your mind and wait patiently for each answer. Maintain curiosity. Allow the answers to emerge intuitively, as your future self "responds." Consider each answer carefully.

4. Travel forward in time and imagine you *are* this other "you." Imagine how life is different, now that you have achieved your goal. What

rewards and satisfactions do you enjoy? Imagine the obstacles you've surmounted and the problems you've solved. Sense the accomplishment! Look backwards to the present. What do you know now that you didn't know then? Imagine looking back at the steps you took. See the milestones. You are "reverse engineering" your goal.

5. Return to the here and now, bringing your discoveries with you. Imagine that, once more, you see your future self, ahead of you in time. This other "you" beckons you to take action and stay motivated. This other "you" is a friend, who is always there with support and encouragement.

6. Reorient and open your eyes.

Another way to create a compelling future is to clearly visualize your outcomes: your new behaviors, thoughts, and emotions that support your goals. You have only to answer a simple question: "What if a miracle happened?"

Self-hypnosis: Visualize Your Outcome with the "Miracle Question"

The late Stephen de Shazer (1940–2005), was an expert in solution-focused behavioral therapy and one of the many therapists influenced by Erickson. De Shazer is credited for the Miracle Question.[44] It is a lead-in to a visualization process that helps you to vividly imagine a future outcome, without having to figure out the preliminary steps, learning, and preparation required. The idea is to "start with the end in mind," and, again, let your unconscious do the reverse engineering to figure out how you arrived at that point. Here is an adaptation of the Miracle Question:

> Imagine that you go to bed tonight and fall into a deep sleep. While you sleep, a miracle occurs! All the resourcefulness, motivation, and commitment needed to accomplish your goal are bestowed upon you. Now pretend it's the following morning. You wake up feeling refreshed and alert. As you proceed through your day, you are consistently demonstrating that the miracle has taken place! What are you doing, thinking, and feeling that is different?

To answer the question, use the self-hypnosis process below. Visualize each answer. See what you would see. Hear what you would hear. Feel the emotions. Take your time with the process. If you don't know an answer, make it up, or better still, let your unconscious present the answer intuitively. Here are the steps:

1. Induce and deepen trance with any method of your choice.

2. Imagine you are beginning your day. Little do you realize that a miracle occurred overnight, but as the day unfolds, you notice what's new and different in your thoughts, emotions, and behaviors. Imagine answers to the questions below:

    - What internal strengths and qualities are you most aware of today?
    - What behaviors are you demonstrating that support your goal?
    - What have you stopped doing? How is it to be free of that behavior?
    - How are your thoughts and emotions changed?
    - What new choices and decisions are you now making?
    - What do others notice? What do they say? How do you respond?
    - What new coping skills are you applying to situations that were previously difficult?
    - How do you feel at the end of the day?

3. Return your thoughts to the here and now. Let the memories of your visualization filter down through your unconscious, settling into every cell, creating a blueprint for future thinking and behavior. Say to yourself, "Yes, that miracle *has* occurred!" Anticipate the changes you'll make as a result, even if you only *pretend* the miracle has occurred.

4. Reorient and open your eyes.

Give yourself permission to believe you can achieve your own miracles. To get any result in life, you have to think of it first – not wistfully, but with purpose and specificity, as you have just done.

Self-Hypnosis: Learn from a Role Model with "Deep Trance Identification"

Role models are people we seek to emulate. Sometimes when striving for a goal or learning a new behavior, we look to others, following their example. Deep trance identification involves a trance-induced identification with a role model.[45] With it, you can learn how to access resources for accomplishing your outcomes. Before you begin, choose someone who demonstrates the kinds of behaviors, emotions, and attitudes you need to accomplish your goal. Here are the steps:

1. Induce and deepen trance using any method of your choice.

2. Visualize a movie of your role model demonstrating the resourceful behaviors that you seek to emulate. Study him carefully to observe nuances and details, such as posture, facial expression, movements, gestures, word choice, pace of speaking, and voice tone.

3. Take the place of your role model. Imagine you *are* him. See with his eyes and hear with his ears. Pretend that you now have access to his thoughts, feelings, values, beliefs, and inner dialog. Where does he get his knowledge? How does he make decisions? You notice things that are useful and instructive. Imagine having his thoughts and actions, understandings and perceptions. Realize what it is to *have* this resourcefulness. Realize what you are now learning. Allow your unconscious mind to absorb whatever is useful and relevant.

4. Guide yourself back into your own mind and body, where you are waiting to receive this knowledge. Allow your unconscious mind to safely integrate this information in a way that is compatible and congruent with your personality, needs, values, and responsibilities. Take all the time you need to complete this integration, making only those changes that are in your best interest.

5. Mental rehearsal: Anticipate a situation in the future when you will accomplish your outcome. Be there now, imagining what you'll see and hear. Imagine that you are accessing a highly resourceful state, demonstrating your desired outcome, with new results. Repeat this mental rehearsal for additional future situations.

6. Bring your thoughts back to the here and now. Reorient and open your eyes.

Make the most of the role models around you. Interview and train with people whom you regard as experts – those who have accomplished goals similar to yours. Read their books. Watch their videos. Learn from a mentor.

What is Your Motivation Strategy?

You've read about several motivation strategies in this chapter. What are your motivation strategies? Think carefully about something you always do, no matter what. What do you tell yourself that makes you do it? What do you visualize? How do you get yourself to do it? How do you feel afterwards? Compare that experience to something you often *want* to do, but you *don't* do it. Again, ask the same questions. How do you *prevent* yourself from doing it? How do you feel afterwards? Identify the critical differences between the two strategies.

For example, when Leanne is motivated to do something, she expects to do it and arranges time for it. She keeps an image in her mind that represents the ultimate value of the task (having money in the bank, maintaining health and fitness, etc.). As the time approaches, she gets ready and tells herself to do it. She imagines doing it, fully associated. This image is followed by two side-by-side associated images. In one, she has completed the task and feels happy and satisfied. In the other, she has avoided the task and feels guilty. Both images make her *want* to do the task. The images represent that she can do the task and feel good about it, and thereby avoid the guilt of not doing it. So she acts on the task, completes it, and feels good afterward.

Conversely, when she *avoids* a task, she has a different strategy. She doesn't plan ahead. When she thinks about doing it, she asks, "Do I want to do this?" Then she realizes she has an option to avoid the task. She makes two side-by-side dissociated images of herself in her mind. In one image, she sees herself doing the task, but having difficulty with it or feeling inconvenienced. In the other image, she sees herself happily doing something else that is easier and more convenient. This second image is larger and more colorful than the other one; much more appealing. Inevitably, Leanne chooses the latter option.

Notice the difference between these two strategies. Can you understand how it is inevitable that she will pursue one task and avoid another? What about *your* strategies for motivation and avoidance? Can you detect the critical differences? Now choose a task that you want to do, but generally avoid. For the next few days, run that task through your mind using your motivation strategy instead of your avoidance strategy. I think you'll discover you feel much more motivated! You'll find two more motivational self-hypnosis strategies in the next chapter.

CHAPTER 12

Stop Procrastinating Once and for All!

To procrastinate is to put something off. To delay or reschedule is a conscious decision, whereas procrastination is a default position, the result of *not* making a decision, *not* taking action, *not* making a commitment, or *not* resolving a problem.

Procrastination is often the result of too much information and feeling overwhelmed with too many choices. At some point, when faced with a decision to act, we simply shut down, push the decision aside, or refuse to think about it. We let things fall through the cracks while we concentrate on whatever seems most urgent or more appealing at the moment.

Procrastination is unfinished business. It plays havoc with priorities, plans, and goals. In a way, it is self-sabotage because the more we put something off, without coming to a clear-cut decision, the higher the penalty.

The costs of procrastination can include late fees, costly repairs when we ignore routine maintenance, poor performance because we don't prepare adequately, missed appointments and opportunities, and health problems that could have been addressed sooner. Sometimes procrastination robs us of time and energy because we keep revisiting the issue or problem, without resolving it. On an interpersonal level, procrastination can affect relationships when we put off responsibilities, keep others waiting for a decision, or fail to meet others' hopes or expectations. On a personal level, procrastination can cause guilt and embarrassment. Procrastination deprives us of something very precious – peace of mind.

Before I introduce you to two self-hypnosis methods for overcoming procrastination, I want to share ten reasons why people procrastinate and what to do about each one.

Ten Common Reasons for Procrastination: What to do about Them

Procrastination is based on a "reason" why we don't take action. If you can identify the reasoning (what you are telling yourself) behind your procrastination, you are more likely to implement the solution. So here are solutions for the most common reasons for procrastination.

Reason 1: The task is too difficult and time-consuming

Stephen Covey wrote that we are most likely to take action on tasks that we regard as urgent.[46] We perceive a task as urgent when *not* doing it carries a consequence. We take care of urgent tasks immediately not because doing so enriches our lives, but because the consequences of ignoring them are too great. We are "putting out fires."

We tend to complete tasks that are easy and convenient, as opposed to those things that are difficult and time-consuming. Ironically, tasks that are most difficult and time-consuming are often those that would, in the long run, most enrich our lives.

Solution: Important tasks usually require careful planning and conscious, concerted effort. Chunk the task down into small, sequential steps and schedule them. Give these steps a high priority. You may need to eliminate other obligations and responsibilities that have a low pay-off value. Purposely set aside time, on a regular basis, to pursue your important tasks. Enlist the support of friends and family.

Reason 2: Improper planning

If you are procrastinating instead of taking action, your plan is faulty in some way. The most common flaws in planning are:

- Insufficient detail: milestones are not broken down into small enough units.
- Tasks are not specific enough to describe the actions you must take.
- Inadequate resources (time, money, personnel, information) or inefficient use of resources.
- Unrealistic target dates, or no target dates, for milestones.
- Lack of planning for contingencies.

- Inflexibility when obstacles arise.

Solution: The solution, of course, is to revise the plan to correct each flaw.

Reason 3: Conflicting priorities

With multiple demands, conflicting priorities are commonplace. We feel pulled in several directions at once. We are faced with the dilemma of addressing some priorities, while procrastinating about others.

Solution: Order your tasks into three categories: A, B, and C.[47] In the A category are those activities that you absolutely will do today. (Hint: If you can't do it in one day, you haven't chunked it down sufficiently.) In the B category are those activities that you will do today, if you complete all the A's. If you don't get the B's done, move them to tomorrow's list. C's are small but generally inconsequential tasks that you'll do if you have time.

Each day, list your priority tasks. Sequence A category tasks, ordering them according to urgency and value. Focus your energies and attention on A level tasks and do them first. Then go on to the B's and C's. (Tip: Let the C's pile up and set aside one day a week to tackle all the C's.)

Reason 4: The task is too small

Some tasks seem so small and insignificant they can be accomplished "any old time," so we put them off because they hardly seem worth the effort. Cleaning up after yourself, putting things back where they belong, sewing on a loose button, emptying the overflowing wastebasket – any of these jobs would take less than 5 minutes. Yet, if we continually procrastinate about the small tasks, eventually they cause problems – like clutter, spills, spoilage, and hazards. Ignoring simple, routine maintenance can result in costly repairs.

Solution: Develop the habit of taking care of small, routine tasks on the spot. Another option is to schedule a "clean-up and catch-up" day, when you block out a few hours of uninterrupted time for tidying, cleaning up, repairing, paperwork, and general housekeeping, maintenance, and administrative tasks.

Reason 5: I don't like it!

We often procrastinate about things we just don't like to do.

Solution: For a task that seems particularly irksome, consider these options:

- Delegate the task or hire someone to do it.

- Barter with a friend or family member to do the task and you do something for him or her in return.

- Eliminate the need to perform the task. If you hate gardening, then pave over your garden and make it into a patio.

- Find a way to make the task tolerable or even enjoyable. Do it to music, do it with a friend, or do it first thing in the morning.

- Maybe you'd enjoy it with better equipment.

- Stop grumbling and revise your self-talk. Instead of telling yourself how miserable you feel, change your dialog to encouragement.

- See the necessity of the task in the context of a larger picture of highly-valued results that make completing the task worthwhile.

- Ask a friend to hold you accountable for finishing the task.

- Plan to give yourself a reward for completing the task. No cheating!

Reason 6: I don't have time

Yes, we are all short on time. Generally, if something matters, you can somehow find the time to do it.

Solution: Hone your time management skills. Read a book or take a class. Learn to identify and eliminate time wasting activities, establish priorities, use time management tools, manage paperwork, delegate, and get organized.

Reason 7: I don't know how!

Sometimes we think we should know how to do a task but we really don't. Instead of confronting the reality and admitting it, we get into denial and procrastinate instead.

Solution: Admit what you don't know and come to terms with it. If the task is important enough, invest time and money to educate yourself. Read a book or take a class. Get a mentor. Hire an expert advisor.

Reason 8: Fear of failure – perfectionism

Some people procrastinate because they fear failure and dread making mistakes. They worry about feeling disappointed or looking foolish in front of others, or about the inconvenience of having to correct mistakes. If we waited until we could do everything perfectly, we'd never do anything! Perfectionism also leads to procrastination when we wait for the perfect moment, the perfect weather, the perfect opportunity, or the perfect tool. Everything must be perfect or we won't do it at all.

Solution: Don't let perfection become the enemy of good enough. A job done well, even though imperfectly, may be better than one not done at all. Realize that mistakes and setbacks are inherent in the process of any significant undertaking. Be willing to make mistakes as you go along, acknowledge them, make corrections, and learn from them. Give yourself permission to be perfectly imperfect.

Reason 9: Indecision

Sometimes we procrastinate because we aren't really sure we want to do the task in the first place. Or maybe we haven't yet decided exactly how we want to do it. Or maybe we can't decide among too many options.

Solution: Look at the advantages and disadvantages of doing the task or not doing it. Get the opinion of others who are involved directly or indirectly. For evaluating several options, compare the advantages and disadvantages of each option.

Reason 10: Hurting someone's feelings

Have you ever put off a difficult decision because it would hurt someone's feelings? It's understandable that your desire to spare someone's feelings would override your desire to resolve an issue. Nevertheless, procrastinating only prolongs your own agonizing. The sooner you resolve the issue, the sooner the injured party can heal, make other arrangements, and move on.

Solution: Speak to the other person honestly and tactfully, without blame. Take full responsibility for your decision, acknowledge the hurt you've caused, and apologize. Offer to make reparations or amends, if possible.

Self-Hypnosis: The NLP Godiva Chocolate Pattern

Richard Bandler developed the NLP Godiva Chocolate Pattern.[48] The purpose of this visualization process is to make your intended outcome seem so irresistible that you absolutely must have it – now! The name comes from the idea that Godiva Chocolate is so appealing, some people find it irresistible. In this pattern, you'll choose something (an object or activity) that you already consistently find so pleasurable, you feel compelled to have it or do it. So choose something irresistible, as long as it is a *positive* in your life. You'll apply this same "must have it/must do it" feeling to your outcome or goal.

Be sure you feel congruent about the outcome you have in mind. This process aims to make your intended outcome *into a compulsion*! Here are the steps:

1. Induce and deepen trance in any way you choose.

2. Image 1: Visualize something you absolutely cannot resist – something you feel wildly compelled to enjoy again and again. Associate into the image. If it's an object, it is right in front of you. If it's an activity, the opportunity to engage in it is immediately available. Let yourself feel the desire, anticipated pleasure, passion, and absolute driving *need* to have or do it.

3. Clear your visual field.

4. Image 2: Make a dissociated image of yourself doing a task you sincerely want to do – a task about which you've been procrastinating. See yourself doing it.

5. Hold Image 2 in mind, with Image 1 behind it. Image 2 hides Image 1, but you know it's there. Open up a tiny hole, like a peephole, in the center of Image 2, so that you can look through that hole to see Image 1.

6. Visualize Image 2. Quickly open up the small hole in the center, so that you instantly see Image 1. Get the full feelings for Image 1.

7. Shrink the hole down quickly, so that you are looking again at Image 2, maintaining the feeling of desire and motivation engendered by Image 1. Let yourself have the feeling that Image 2 is irresistible, enjoyable, and appealing. You have to do it!

8. Repeat Steps 6 and 7, three to five more times, as quickly as you can. Each time, visualize Image 2, peep through to Image 1, get the feelings from Image 1, close the peephole, and transfer the feelings to Image 2.

9. Clear your visual field. Visualize Image 2, without the peephole, and notice how much more motivated you feel for Image 2.

10. Mental rehearsal: Associate fully into Image 2, visualizing how you'll consistently take action on your outcome, feeling completely motivated!

11. Return your thoughts to the here and now. Reorient and open your eyes.

Self-Hypnosis: Get into Action with the Mind-to-Muscle Pattern

The Mind-to-Muscle Pattern is a motivation strategy that chains a series of thoughts into a pattern for taking action. It was developed by L. Michael Hall to help you bridge the gap between understanding what you want to do and actually doing it.[49]

Identify any task that you already perform routinely and without fail. It might be going to work, tucking your children in at night, or feeding your cat. These are habits. You expect to do them without reminding, coaxing, or arguing yourself into it. You could say, then, that a habit is a mind-to-muscle connection. Hall wrote:

> Ultimately, personal mastery arises from the ability to turn highly ... valued principles into *neurological patterns*. As with typing ... the original learning may take a considerable

amount of time and trouble in order to get the muscle patterns and coordination deeply imprinted. Yet once we have practiced and trained ... then *the learnings become incorporated into the very fabric of the muscles themselves* ... At that point we have translated *principle into muscle*. (Hall, 2000, p. 238; italics in original)

The Mind-to-Muscle Pattern converts thought into muscle, so you actually feel the need to act on your outcome. In this chain-like process, you move from understanding to belief, decision, and action. You can do this pattern with your eyes open or closed. Read it over and journal on it first or discuss it aloud with yourself or a friend before actually doing it. Here are the steps:

1. Induce and deepen trance with any method of your choice.

2. Identify a principle associated with your outcome. What do you understand that makes your intended outcome worth the effort? Putting it another way, what is the value and/or meaning that makes you want this outcome? Why do it at all? Make your principle into a sentence: "I understand that ..." (Example: "I understand that exercise will give me good health and stamina.")

3. Describe the principle as a belief. Make the belief into a sentence: "I firmly believe that ..." (Example: "I firmly believe that a healthy body is the supreme instrument of life!"). Say it convincingly to yourself.

4. Reformat the belief as a decision, expressed as a sentence that begins, "I choose to ..." (Example: "I choose to exercise regularly.") Say this sentence convincingly and congruently to yourself. Let your feelings match the words.

5. Rephrase the decision as a mind–body state: "With my decision to ... I feel ... and I experience ..." (Example: "With my decision to exercise, I feel empowered, and I see myself getting strong and healthy.")

6. State the action you intend as an expression of the above steps: "The one thing I will do today as an expression of my belief, my decision, and my feelings, is ..." Finish that sentence and say, with sincere conviction, what you will do – your next action toward your goal.

7. Mental rehearsal: Visualize the action you will take today. Associate fully into the image, seeing what you would see, hearing what you would hear. Imagine doing it.

8. Mental rehearsal while going "meta": Keep visualizing your action. Feel the motivation. Restate your decision with a full awareness of how your decision empowers your ability to take action. Say a powerful "Yes!" to your decision. Restate your belief, as now exemplified by your action. Say a powerful "Yes!" to that belief. Restate the understandings that now drive home a clear rationale for your action. Yes! Restate your belief even more powerfully. Yes! Restate your decision even more convincingly. Yes! Restate your feelings and really experience them. Yes!

9. Repeat Step 8 three to five times until your motivation feels unstoppable!

10. Return your thoughts to the here and now. Arrange to take action. Anticipate the actions you'll continue to exert until your goal is accomplished. Visualize your ultimate goal, waiting in your future. Reorient and open your eyes.

The Mind-to-Muscle Pattern forms an emotional attachment to your outcome by associating it to a belief. When you believe in something completely, you act on your belief, do you not?

What Do You Deserve?

Procrastination is a form of self-sabotage when we keep ourselves from accomplishing the outcomes we most want. In *Stop Self-Sabotage!* Pat Pearson, a psychotherapist and motivational speaker (no relation to me), wrote that we sometimes sabotage ourselves and put off achieving our goals because, unconsciously, we believe that we don't deserve these things.[50] Such beliefs can often be traced back to things we learned in childhood – what others told us and what we observed in others.

You can take steps to increase feelings of deserving. The steps are:

- Confront the negative things you say to yourself and the negative beliefs you hold. Determine to release these beliefs. See Chapter 16 for a self-hypnosis remedy for limiting beliefs about yourself.

- Confront negative feelings, such as unresolved grief and anger, and work to release them. You can do this through talking to a therapist or counselor, joining a support group, or speaking frankly with those who have wronged you.

- Change your self-talk to focus not on your limitations but on life-affirming goals.

- Give yourself permission to accomplish the goals you envision.

- Nurture yourself even when you experience setbacks and make mistakes.

- Create an emotional support system of friends who can applaud your successes and give you help and encouragement.

Believe that your life has intrinsic value. Everyone has a dream they want to realize. What's yours? How will you accomplish it?

CHAPTER 13

Improve Your Performance

Self-hypnosis has long enjoyed a reputation among top athletes, performers, sales people, public speakers, and executives as a primary secret behind their success. They might call it meditation, visualization, or mental practice – it's all a form of self-hypnosis; a way of preparing to meet challenges and excel. The essential feature is an image of oneself as confident, competent, and successful in achieving an outcome. This chapter will serve as a guide for bringing about your best performance in a wide range of endeavors. In this chapter you'll learn self-hypnosis strategies to:

- Access optimum confidence.
- Achieve your personal best in sports.
- Acquire a strategy to recover quickly from mistakes.
- Respond resourcefully to criticism.

I chose the first item on the list – optimum confidence – because, when it comes to performance, it is the most frequent request that I get in my practice. Most people want to feel confident any time they present themselves or perform in front of others. The second item, achieving personal best in sports, is something I often teach young athletes. The next two items, recovering from mistakes and responding resourcefully to criticism, are most appropriate for improved performance in sports, the performing arts, and in the workplace.

Tips for Abolishing Performance Anxiety

All of us, I believe, want our talents to shine in the eyes of those around us. We want to win the good opinions and good will of others. Sometimes, however, we fear mistakes and the unfavorable judgments of others to the extent that we develop performance anxiety. This is often an expression of the desire to perform well which, paradoxically, makes it impossible to perform well. We place such a high premium on a perfect performance that instead of activating confidence, we activate fear – fear of failure, fear of embarrassment, fear of rejection by others. That fear triggers anxiety. It's impossible feel anxiety and confidence at the same time.

It's not a pretty picture. It gets even worse if you berate yourself for *having* anxiety. You may have discovered that berating yourself does not make you feel more confident. It only triggers the fear centers in the brain which, in turn, activates the autonomic nervous system, bringing about more anxiety, and increases the likelihood of making mistakes.

In Chapter 4 you read about the value of mental rehearsal. Almost all the self-hypnosis strategies in this book rely on mental rehearsal, so that the behavioral changes you see in your mind become the behaviors you exhibit in real life. Mental rehearsal works wonderfully for improved performance. Sadly, those with performance anxiety use mental rehearsal the wrong way – and they do it unwittingly. They envision everything that could go wrong! They envision humiliation and blunders. They create a self-fulfilling prophecy because they keep mentally rehearsing what they most want to avoid.

Here are a few tips for overcoming performance anxiety.

- **Practice.** Practice your performance. Don't expect perfection in the beginning. Each mistake you make in practice is one less mistake you'll make when the curtain rises or when you enter the arena of competition. When you practice, use "helps" until you master the moves you want. Practice in front of a mirror. Roleplay with a trusted friend. Follow diagrams, storyboards, flowcharts, notecards, a training video or whatever will facilitate memory and coordination. Practice with a coach who can guide you, encourage you, and tell you how to improve.

- **Realize it's not about you.** When you perform for others, stop thinking about yourself. Think about the gift that you are giving to others around you. Think about giving your audience, your colleagues, your team members the gift of your knowledge, talent, and skill. Get your mind off yourself. Stop feeling like a victim. You've got something worthwhile to share.

- **Stop dwelling on past mistakes and failures.** Learn from the past and move on. The reason people dwell on their past mistakes is because they worry that those mistakes will happen again. They want to prevent a repeat of a bad memory. But dwelling on the past does not make for improvement. The key to success is to apply what you learned and focus on what you are now doing differently. Don't let a past mistake determine how you perform today and in the future.

- **Have a healthy approach.** For excellent performance, and for any type of competition, take care of yourself health-wise. Get adequate sleep, good nutrition, and exercise. Don't try to get your confidence from drugs or alcohol – you'll regret it in the long run. With a healthy approach, you'll have the energy and mental clarity that make for a winner.

- **Take time with your appearance.** Let's face it, when you look good, you feel good. Maybe looks shouldn't matter as much as they do, and sure, millionaire Steve Jobs could afford to take to the stage in his blue jeans. However, unless you are already rich and famous, sprucing up won't hurt. Send your suit to the cleaners, get a haircut, and shine your shoes. When it comes to an audition, a job interview, a sales call, or a speaking appearance, you'll feel more confident and your audience will be much more favorably impressed with you if you look the part.

Self-Hypnosis: Access Optimum Confidence with the NLP Circle of Excellence

As an NLP trainer, I've witnessed many variations on the Circle of Excellence. This NLP pattern is so easy, even school-aged children can learn it – and they often do so with pleasure and glee. I especially like this pattern because it is a variation on anchoring that you can learn standing on your feet.

Initially you'll complete the three steps of the pattern standing up. Then you can review the pattern in trance. I'll give separate instructions on the mental rehearsal step for specific applications: public speaking, a job interview, an audition or stage performance, or introducing yourself to others at a social event. Vary these examples to your needs. If you have another application in which you want optimum confidence, make up your own mental rehearsal. Just include sufficient detail, as you'll see in my examples, to make your rehearsal vivid and realistic.

To learn the three steps of the NLP Circle of Excellence, stand up. On the floor in front of you, imagine a row of three circles, side by side, each the size of a hula-hoop. We'll number these circles, 1, 2 and 3. Circle 1 represents a past experience, in which you'll anchor a state of confidence. Circle 2 represents the here and now, in which you intensify that state. Circle 3 represents a future experience, in which you mentally rehearse optimum confidence.

- Step into Circle 1, accessing a vivid memory of a past experience in which you felt optimum confidence. It can be any context, even one unrelated to your outcome. Associate to the experience. Imagine that you are really there, right now. See what you saw. Hear what you heard. Revivify the feelings of confidence!

- Holding on to the confident feelings, step into Circle 2, into the here and now. Using all your senses, intensify that state of confidence. Alter your posture and your facial expression to show your confidence. Breathe in deeply, imagining that you are breathing in the energy of confidence. Feel the confidence from head to toe. Imagine some sound, like music, applause, or cheering, which amplifies your confident feelings. Taste and smell confidence. Let the confident feelings move out around you into your energy field. Visualize your confidence glowing and sparkling about you like an aura. Say aloud, convincingly, "Yes! I feel confident! I speak confidently. I move confidently through the world. I think confidently about my abilities and skills."

- Step into Circle 3, visualizing that you are stepping into a future challenge or opportunity. Bring the confidence with you as you step into this circle. Holding on to that feeling of confidence, mentally rehearse how you'll behave in that situation.

Here are a few examples of what you can imagine in Circle 3:

- **Public speaking:** You are standing in front of a room of people and speaking confidently. Own the platform and command the listeners' attention. Welcome your moment in the spotlight. Remember: this isn't about you; it's about your message. You have something to say, so say it loud and clear! Your heartbeat is steady. You breathe freely and easily. Your gestures are smooth and natural. Your posture shows that you feel composed and at ease. You make eye contact with individuals in your audience, focusing on friendly faces. You speak clearly and audibly, with a pace that suits your message. Your thoughts are organized. You easily remember what you intend to say and how to say it. You appreciate that others are listening.

- **A job interview:** You shake hands with your interviewer when you meet her. You say a few pleasantries, feeling confident, alert, and friendly. You walk confidently to the interview room. You sit in the chair with a comfortable, confident posture. You get into rapport with the interviewer, following her lead in terms of postures, gestures, and pacing the conversation. You answer questions sincerely, with self-assurance. You convey that you are a competent, skilled candidate for the job, who can solve problems. When you speak, your voice is clear and audible. You know just what to say. Your heartbeat is steady. You breathe freely and easily. You look the interviewer in the eye. You ask a few questions of your own to demonstrate your interest in the company.

- **An audition or stage performance:** When you walk out on stage, believe that this stage now belongs to you. The moment is magical! You are fully immersed in your performance, with keen concentration. You have prepared and now that preparation pays dividends! Your memory for every nuance is superb. You feel confident as you say your lines, act the part, sing, perform, and/or demonstrate your skills. Your heartbeat is steady. You breathe freely and easily. You possess a commanding presence. Your voice comes out in the just the way you want it to. Your gestures are natural and fluid. Your posture is perfect for the occasion. A positive, electric energy is flowing all around you and through you.

- **Introducing yourself to others at a social event:** As you walk into the event, you feel energized, friendly, and confident. You say to yourself, "I like people and people like me!" You look around and find someone to talk to. You stride confidently toward that individual with a friendly expression. You breathe freely and easily. You introduce yourself, extending your right hand. "Hello, my name is … I notice that you …" Finish this sentence with a compliment or a kindness. Example: "I notice that you have a lovely ring – I've never seen one like it," or "I notice that you haven't yet been to the buffet. I haven't either. Would you like to walk there with me?" You speak confidently and you look people in the eye. Your handshake conveys sincerity. You listen attentively to others. You ask follow-up questions about what they say. You smile frequently. You make smooth transitions as you move from person to person or from small group to small group. You enjoy meeting so many fascinating individuals!

The second phase is the self-hypnosis phase. Find a comfortable place to sit or recline. Follow these steps:

1. Induce and deepen trance with any method of your choosing.

2. Revivify your experience in Circle 1.Visualize the memory again, in detail, bringing back all those feelings of confidence.

3. Holding on to those feelings of confidence, visualize, once more, that you are stepping into Circle 2. Once more, intensify the feelings of confidence in the here and now.

4. Mental rehearsal: Visualize stepping to Circle 3. Holding on to those feelings of confidence, imagine a future performance in which you feel confident. Visualize the details: your movements, posture, breathing, thoughts, feelings, self-talk, facial expressions, voice, and actions.

5. Reorient and open your eyes.

Self-Hypnosis: Achieve Your Personal Best in Sports

Sports psychology is the application of psychological principles and methods to help athletes improve their performance by sharpening their "mental game." Sports psychologists use hypnotherapy and teach athletes self-hypnosis for a wide variety of applications.[51] I've listed a few such uses below, with chapter references where you can find relevant information on self-hypnosis methods. If you are an athlete, you can use self-hypnosis to:

- Make sure you sleep well on the night before competition (see Chapter 9).

- Visualize a goal (e.g., winning a championship) (see Goal Imaging in Chapter 4).

- Feel motivated to practice (see Chapter 11).

- Manage pain from sports injuries (see Chapter 17).

- Emulate a favorite sports figure (see Self-Hypnosis: Learn from a Role Model with "Deep Trance Identification" in Chapter 11).

- Access maximum confidence (in addition to Self-Hypnosis: NLP Circle of Excellence in this chapter, see Self-Hypnosis: A Resourceful Self-Image in the introduction to Part II).

- Quickly recover from a mistake and regain focus (see Self-Hypnosis: Recover Quickly from Mistakes, later in this chapter).

- Cope effectively with criticism (see Self-Hypnosis: NLP Responding Resourcefully to Criticism Pattern, later in this chapter).

Now we turn to self-hypnosis for peak performance. When athletes play especially well, they are in "the zone" – a state of heightened awareness and concentration, where movement and coordination take on a fluidity that makes performance effortless. The zone usually occurs only when an athlete has practiced extensively and thoroughly developed the neural nets that support optimum movement and coordination. The zone is an eyes-open trance state that usually happens by chance. However, you can condition your mind to access that state more easily, more often, with self-hypnosis.

Here are the steps:

1. Induce and deepen trance with any method of your choosing.

2. Recall a moment in the past where you were in the zone in your sport. Associate into this experience. Be there. Relive the sights, sounds, motion, smells, and emotions. Immerse yourself completely in this memory.

3. Imagine that your neurological structures are recording and memorizing everything about your state in Step 2. Anchor this experience with a tactile cue such as tapping your elbow three times in quick succession.

4. Repeat Steps 2 and 3 three to five more times until your mind and body are making a reliable association between your anchored cue (e.g., tapping your elbow) and accessing the zone.

5. Return your thoughts to the here and now. Test your anchor. Tap your elbow three times (or activate whatever cue you've chosen) and feel yourself accessing the zone. Notice now that you can easily get into the zone. You also want to exit the zone at will. So change your posture or alter your breathing in such a way that you easily exit the zone.

6. Mental rehearsal: Visualize participating in an upcoming event in your sport. Imagine you are there now, getting involved in the action. Apply your cue to access the zone. Imagine playing your game in the zone.

7. Give yourself the suggestion: When I play (name your sport) I play in the zone. Return your thoughts to the here and now. Reorient and open your eyes.

Self-Hypnosis: Recover Quickly from Mistakes

Are you someone who feels confident most of the time until you make a mistake – and then your confidence wilts? Mistakes are especially difficult when they happen in front of others. We feel awkward and embarrassed, wanting to crawl into a hole. Mistakes can throw off mental and physical performance – *unless* you have a recovery strategy.

Many years ago I read about a study conducted with a class of college students. The students were told they would have a guest instructor that day. The instructor was actually part of a research experiment. She waited until the students were in their seats and entered the classroom, carrying a load of books and papers. Upon entering, she "accidentally" dropped her papers, scattering them on the floor. As she picked them up, she apologized, made self-effacing remarks, and acted embarrassed. Then she proceeded to give a short lecture, said goodbye, and left the classroom.

The same experiment was then carried out with a second classroom. However, in the second classroom, when the instructor dropped her books and papers, she calmly picked them up, without apologizing, making self-effacing remarks, or acting embarrassed. She then proceeded to give the same short lecture, say goodbye, and leave the classroom.

The same two versions of the experiment took place in multiple classrooms. The students were then asked to rate the instructor's effectiveness. When she did not act embarrassed, she received higher ratings. The research suggested that the students saw the instructor as more competent when she did not get flustered by her "mistake."

Mistakes are inevitable. The ability to quickly recover from them will improve your performance and your ability to refocus on the task at hand. It might also boost your competence in others' eyes. The secret to recovering quickly is to acknowledge a mistake, regard the mistake as feedback, make any necessary adjustments in your behavior, and refocus. The self-hypnosis session below will help. Here are the steps:

1. Induce and deepen trance with any method of your choice.

2. Recall a time when you made a mistake and felt flustered, anxious, or embarrassed by it. Briefly recall what happened and how you felt.

3. Return your thoughts to the here and now. Take a few deep breaths to release the discomfort of that memory. Return to feeling calm and relaxed.

4. Visualize a movie of yourself making the mistake. Remember, this is a dissociated image. Stop the movie just one second after the "you" in the movie makes the mistake. Now change the scenario. This time, visualize that this other "you" immediately acknowledges the mistake, "Oops! I just made a mistake."

Next, this other "you" reviews the mistake one time, with the question, "How shall I correct that mistake and get back on task?" This other "you" then quickly makes any necessary corrections or adjustments. Next, this other "you" says, "That mistake is over and done. I put it behind me." Watch as this other "you" refocuses on the task at hand, moving back into task-oriented behavior.

Reach out with your arms and pull this other "you" into your body, so that you are integrating this new strategy into your repertoire.

5. Return to the scene in Step 2. Be there, but play it through this time with your new strategy. Make the mistake, pause, review, and ask, "How shall I correct that mistake and get back on task?" Visualize that you are making any necessary corrections or adjustments. Say to yourself, "That mistake is over and done. I put it behind me." Visualize that you refocus on the task at hand and resume action.

6. Practice Step 5 three to five times until you have memorized the sequence.

7. Affirmation: I recover easily from mistakes and move on with improved performance.

8. Return your thoughts to the here and now. Anticipate that you'll apply this strategy in the future when you make a mistake. Reorient and open your eyes.

You can't predict when or where your next mistake will occur. When it does, you'll be ready with this strategy. If someone criticizes your mistake, or you learn about your mistake through someone's criticism, the next section will help you to cope constructively with criticism.

Self-Hypnosis: NLP Responding Resourcefully to Criticism Pattern

At one time or another, we've all had difficulty with responding to criticism. Some people instantly feel anxious when criticized. They either beat up on themselves or get angry and defend themselves. Either way, they usually make a bad situation worse and they block out information, some of which may be useful.

To respond resourcefully to criticism is to treat criticism as information. With such information, you might improve your performance or avoid a future pitfall – or you might decide to do nothing with it at all. You can make a clear-headed decision about what to do with criticism only if you examine the content objectively.

When someone criticizes you rudely or harshly, refuse to take it personally. Instead, take it as a sign that the person criticizing is not communicating skillfully at that moment. You might actually disarm him by applauding his ability to speak up, even if you disagree with the message. You might calm her emotions by agreeing with the parts of the criticism that seem valid and negotiating the other parts. By staying calm and detached, you can ask clarifying questions, rather than getting defensive.

The NLP Responding Resourcefully to Criticism Pattern (developed by Connirae and Steve Andreas) will help you to stay calm and collected in the face of criticism, while you regard it as information that may or may not be useful.[52] The strategy is to actually *hear* the information, ask clarifying questions, evaluate the validity of the information, and decide whether you want to act on the information by demonstrating different behavior in the future. The essential feature of the strategy is to stay dissociated while evaluating the criticism. Once you learn the steps of this strategy in self-hypnosis, you can apply it easily and instantly in real-life situations.

Here are the steps:

1. Access and deepen trance with any method of your choice.

2. Briefly remember a time when you were criticized and you responded with emotional discomfort. Access the memory just long enough to remember what happened and how it felt.

3. Return your thoughts to the here and now. Take a few deep breaths to release the discomfort of that memory. Return to feeling calm and relaxed.

4. Visualize that you are watching a movie of yourself receiving that criticism. Remember: this is a *dissociated* image. Imagine how this other "you" – the one in the movie – could respond to the criticism in a different way, as follows:

    - See the other "you" receiving the criticism.

    - Imagine that the "you" in the movie calmly and objectively evaluates the criticism. See that this other "you" visualizes the words, themselves, as though they are floating in the air in a "thought balloon."

    - Pretend you can hear the thoughts of this other "you" as he calmly asks himself questions about the words: "Is this person a trustworthy source for this information? Is there anything valid in this information? Is there anything useful here?"

    - Watch the "you" in the movie make another thought balloon, visualizing in that thought balloon a picture of himself doing what the critic has described. This other "you" evaluates his own imagery, in the thought balloon, to decide if the criticism is valid. This other version of "you" compares what he sees in the balloon with what he knows about his own behavior. Maybe there's a match, maybe not. Perhaps this other "you" needs more information to decide.

    - Now watch the thought balloons disappear, as this other "you" decides what to do with the information. Watch how this other "you" responds resourcefully to the person who delivered the criticism.

5. Appreciate that the "you" in the movie has a new strategy. Reach out with your arms and pull him into your body, integrating this strategy into your repertoire.

6. Affirmation: I regard criticism as potentially useful information.

7. Mental rehearsal: Imagine a possible future scenario involving criticism. You receive the criticism, visualize the words, and ask yourself questions about the words. Then make a dissociated image of the content of the criticism. Compare the image content to what you know about your own behavior. Is the criticism valid? Does it contain useful information? If so, what do you want to do with that information? Imagine how you could respond effectively to the person delivering the criticism.

   Practice on several future scenarios. If you encounter anything that you find difficult, first watch a movie of yourself responding to the criticism, using the above strategy. Then mentally practice your response a second time in an associated manner.

• Bring your thoughts back to the here and now and reorient.

No one is universally loved and adored. There is no law saying that people *shouldn't* criticize you. In fact, if someone does, it could mean you've succeeded in reaching a point at which people notice what you do and form opinions about it. People who receive the most criticism are often those who have reached the pinnacle of their careers.

There's no law that you should feel wronged by someone's criticism or take it as a negative reflection on your worthiness. Anyone can make mistakes, offend another, or perform poorly once in a while. If the criticism is deserved, acknowledge the error and follow the strategy for recovering quickly from mistakes in the previous section of this chapter. Even if you've made a mistake, exercised poor judgment, or performed poorly, you aren't required to feel bad about it indefinitely. Feeling bad about it for five minutes is much more efficient than feeling bad about it for five days. If you can process the information in minutes, why take days feeling bad about it?

The NLP Success Formula

NLP offers a five-step formula for success that will improve any performance you choose.

1. **Know your outcome.** You've read about the well-formed outcome in Chapter 3. To know your outcome is to have evidence-based criteria that will tell you when you have achieved it. Know your outcome so well that you can visualize it and describe it.

2. **Take action toward your outcome.** Develop a plan and act on your plan. Without action, goals and plans are worthless.

3. **Have the sensory acuity to notice whether or not you are getting your outcome.** Confidence is great – as long as you are proceeding confidently in the right direction! If your plan involves a complex project, then set milestones that will help you evaluate the direction of your progress. Be open to feedback, both internal and external.

4. **Have the behavioral flexibility to alter your behavior if what you are doing isn't getting you closer to your outcome.** The truly great accomplishments are usually made by people who keep experimenting and learning from mistakes until they get it right.

5. **Operate from a physiology and a psychology of excellence.** This requires that you operate, physically, from health, stamina, and vitality. Keeping your body in optimum physical condition will contribute to a successful performance in any endeavor. This step also requires that you perform mentally and emotionally from a resourceful state. Successful performance requires the best you can offer from body and mind.

CHAPTER 14

Pass Your Polygraph Exam

Years ago, I held a position requiring a security clearance. Periodically, like all the other employees at the firm where I worked, I had to take a polygraph exam. My colleagues faced the exam with dread and foreboding, agonizing days beforehand. Many spent over an hour in the examiner's office. Over half "failed" and had to retake the exam two or three times. Everyone was very surprised when I was in and out of the exam in 15 minutes, having passed easily. When people asked me how I did it, I simply smiled. Only one or two close friends instantly guessed that I had relied on self-hypnosis – oh, and of course, telling the truth.

Does your job security depend on your ability to pass a polygraph exam? Increasingly, corporations, small businesses, and government agencies require employees in positions of trust to undergo polygraph examinations. The exam consists of a few non-invasive physiological measures of heart rate, blood pressure, and galvanic skin response. You might have a heart monitor strapped around your chest, a blood pressure cuff on your arm, and two small metal plates attached to your finger. It is not physically uncomfortable. Moreover, examiners are trained to be professional and courteous.

Nevertheless, many people are intimidated by the exam. When an examinee feels nervous, it's harder for the examiner to get an accurate reading. This means that even when you are telling the truth, and you've done nothing wrong, your readout might suggest otherwise. Why? Because the polygraph isn't a measure of truth. It's a measure of anxiety.

Most people in positions of trust are honest, decent, and trustworthy with nothing to hide. So why do so many feel anxious about the polygraph exam? They feel anxious about the exam because they perceive that their credibility and often their job security are riding on the results! They worry that they will have to reveal some embarrassing or shameful secret of their past. They get anxious about getting anxious! Their anxiety causes the very results they want to avoid! However, there is a solution. Any honest, truthful person can pass a polygraph easily, with a simple self-hypnosis tactic.

Bear in mind that I'm not siding with criminals or cheats. I do not suggest for one second that anyone should lie or cover up facts during a polygraph exam. In fact, I think everyone should tell the absolute truth. If you are doing something dishonest or illegal, chances are you'll get caught anyway. You might as well confess and face the consequences. I'm on the side of honest people who just want to keep their jobs. To those people I'm saying: if you can control your anxiety, you can stop worrying about your polygraph exam.

What You Need to Know about the Polygraph

Polygraph examiners are trained to convince you that they can detect, from your physiological responses, whether you are lying or telling the truth. They first ask simple questions that anyone can easily answer truthfully – your name, your address, and so on. Your physical readout provides a baseline. Then the examiner asks you to lie purposely, to get a reading on your "lie." After that, any answer you give with the same readout will be deemed a "lie" or at least questionable.

The problem is this: you can tell the truth and still feel anxious about the answer because some of the questions are designed to stir up guilt. They are questions such as "Have you ever stolen anything?" Of course! Everyone has stolen *something*! Do you tell that you stole a cookie from a classmate in first grade? Yes, if that's what comes to mind. But wait! That isn't what the examiner is looking for!

The examiner wants to know if you've ever stolen from an employer, for example. So now you search your conscience trying to cooperate and dredge up the slightest offense – did you accidentally take your supervisor's pen and forget to return it? What about that paper clip? To guide you to the right answer, your unconscious mind helps out by producing feelings of guilt. We are conditioned to associate guilt with anxiety because of the fear of punishment. For many people, even if they haven't done anything wrong, just talking about wrongdoing or thinking about it can bring up anxious feelings.

Ooops! Now the needles on the polygraph are bouncing all over the place – and you are "caught" in the act of "lying!" You are floundering and, realizing that the examiner suspects you are lying, you feel even more anxious. The readout says surely you've stolen something and since you can't say what it is, you could be covering up. You won't "pass" that question!

The irony about the polygraph is that there have been some cases where really dishonest people have passed with flying colors! Why? Because they have no guilt about their nefarious activities or about lying, so they lie with impunity. That's why sometimes a dishonest person can fool a polygraph, while the honest person fails.

Nevertheless, you can maintain a conscience and still pass a polygraph exam. You can make the examiner's job easier if you relax and give an honest answer: "Nothing immediately comes to mind." The examiner would like to get on with his day as much as you would. He isn't your enemy and he isn't there to make you feel miserable. *You* are making *yourself* miserable! He is just doing his job. His job is to ask the questions. Your job is to answer in a way that allows the examiner to see an "honest" readout.

You can give an "honest" readout by telling the truth and by maintaining a detached, calm state in which your heartbeat, pulse rate, body temperature, and blood pressure are normal and natural. The secret to passing a polygraph is to realize that a polygraph exam is not therapy. You don't have to bear your soul. You just have to keep your mind and physical responses under control long enough to give an "honest" readout.

Self-Hypnosis: Pass Your Polygraph Exam Feeling Calm and Detached

You can practice this self-hypnosis method ahead of time, and then apply it in the polygraph room. Here are the steps:

1. Let your body relax completely from head to toe. The polygraph examiner will hook up the devices and explain procedures to you. Listen and cooperate. Ask any questions you need to for clarification of the instructions.

2. When the examiner says that the examination will begin, without needing to close your eyes, let your brain slip into alpha. If you've been practicing the inductions in Chapter 5, you should easily reach alpha frequency, maintaining an eyes-open trance. Relax your body and steady your breathing.

3. Choose an object (not the polygraph machine!) in the room within your range of vision and focus your attention on it. It could even be your own foot or hand. Let your attention be absolutely absorbed by the object. Study it carefully, noticing every detail. Keep your thoughts solely in the present, concentrating on the object. Don't analyze yourself or the examination process. Keep your thoughts in the here and now.

    An advanced method is to mentally dissociate from your body, while concentrating on the object. To dissociate means that you imagine stepping outside of yourself and visualize watching yourself, while you continue to concentrate on the object.

4. The examiner will ask questions. Answer each one calmly, truthfully, and succinctly. Do not elaborate unless you are asked to do so. Don't search through your past for obscure examples of wrongdoing. Keep your thoughts glued to the present. If the examiner presses you to remember something, say, "Nothing comes to mind right now." If you think of some wrongdoing, go ahead and admit it. Chances are it was so innocuous that it isn't likely to jeopardize your job anyway.

Remember, these instructions are for people who are innocent and trustworthy. Keep pulling your thoughts back into the present.

5. The examiner may make some indication that things are not going well. He might sigh heavily, fiddle with the machinery, repeat questions, or say "Hmmm!" He may be genuinely concerned about an inconclusive reading, or it may be just a tactic to make you feel ill at ease. Ignore it. He might even leave the room, so as to observe what you do next through a hidden camera or a two-way mirror. Stay relaxed and keep focusing on your object. Keep your thoughts in the present. Think only pleasant thoughts.

6. Continue until the end of the exam.

The object of this method is to help you (1) maintain a relaxed body state, (2) choose a point of focus, and (3) remain present in the moment. The third item, "remain present in the moment" is important, so that your mind doesn't wander into the past looking for some wrongdoing with which you can "incriminate" yourself. Follow these instructions and you improve your chances of passing the exam.

CHAPTER 15

Give Your Self-Esteem a Lift!

You weren't born with high or low self-esteem. As a baby, you had no sense of guilt, shame, or embarrassment. You were perfectly happy to run around naked, fill your diapers, smear food on your face, and belch in front of others. You screamed if your needs weren't met. You slept whenever you wanted to. Then, through socialization and enculturation, you learned to evaluate and judge yourself and compare yourself to others.

Self-esteem is a *learned* belief about self. How you feel about yourself is a matter of what you were taught. Unfortunately, some children are taught that mistakes and misbehaviors are a cause for shame and possibly the withdrawal of love and approval. They acquire shame-based beliefs about worthiness, competence, and lovability. These beliefs translate to:

- I'm a defective human being.
- I don't deserve to be happy.
- I'm not worthy of my desires.
- I can't do anything right.
- No decent individual could ever possibly love me.

Where does self-esteem come from? Psychotherapist and life coach, Brock Hansen, wrote a book about socialization and parenting called *Shame and Anger: The Criticism Connection.*[53] He suggested that societies and families use criticism, shame, disapproval, and punishment to uphold social standards and promote conformity.

Through shame and conformity we develop a conscience. We understand right from wrong. We distinguish the socially acceptable from the unacceptable. However, when shame is reinforced by trauma and abuse (physical or psychological), then shame becomes toxic. Toxic shame leads to emotional and behavioral disorders as well an erosion of self-esteem. With toxic shame, people learn to evaluate their worth and acquire their sense of self through others' opinions. Through toxic shame, people evaluate themselves as unworthy, defective and inadequate, unable to meet standards, and incapable of finding lasting love, success, or personal happiness. Even when basking in the limelight, they feel like imposters.

Toxic Shame Creates Low Self-Esteem

Toxic shame leads to a learned belief that one is not good enough. Here is the toxic shame strategy for low self-esteem:

1. Think about something you want to have, do, or become.
2. Compare yourself to others who more skilled, accomplished, or fortunate.
3. Feel inadequate by comparison. Criticize, blame, and berate yourself for your perceived inadequacies.
4. Feel anxious, sad, or depressed.
5. Avoid situations that might expose your weaknesses or inadequacies.
6. Don't get what you want to have, do, or become.
7. Start over.

How depressing! Is there a remedy for low self-esteem? Yes! First, develop a philosophy of loving who you are.

A Philosophy of Loving Who You Are

Here are a few philosophical guidelines for living with the one person you can never leave – yourself. Since you have no choice but to be you, and to live in your own skin 24 hours a day for your entire life, you might as well have a philosophy that allows you to love who you are. The first three items in this philosophy are relatively easy. The remainder follow in no particular order, and they are much bigger undertakings.

- Make a conscious decision to love and respect yourself. Commit to creating your best life and your best health. Change what you can and accept what you cannot.

- Believe it's acceptable to love yourself, simply because you are you. No one is perfect and you don't have to be either. How is disliking yourself going to make you a better person?

- Stop comparing yourself to others. Because of individual uniqueness, comparisons are meaningless as a way of determining self-worth. If you see another whom you admire, choose that person as a role model. Instead of comparing yourself to others, strive for your personal best.

- Pursue your passions and life purpose, regardless of what others may do or think. My friend, NLP trainer and life coach, Carol Goldsmith, produced a charming book called *The Book of Carols*, in which she shared her most valued life lessons.[54] She wrote that she purchased a book by an author whom she both envied and admired. She attended a seminar by the author and asked her to sign the book. Two months later, Carol learned that the author had died, unexpectedly, of a brain aneurism, in her thirties. Carol looked again at the inscription inside the book cover. It read, "Carol – Make your life matter. J." Reflecting on this, Carol wrote:

  > Every life matters. Every one of us has a special purpose for our limited time here on Earth, something we know we are destined to do. Maybe it's writing a book, raising a family, starting a business, teaching a class, encouraging others to be their best ... The question is: How do you know? How do you know if that little voice in the back of your head, that quiver of excitement in your belly or chest, that flush of admiration and envy you feel when another person takes center stage, is an indicator of what you should do with your life? Could it be your intuition ... telling you what matters most? There's only one way you'll ever find out. Just go for it."(Goldsmith, 2003, p. 166)

- Map your life journey – make a plan and set objectives. Chart milestones. If you aren't sure how to proceed, don't get discouraged – get curious. Ask questions and search for answers. Behold your potential and decide how you want to define your life. Take a class, read a book, get a mentor, hire a coach. Knowledge is meant to be shared, taught, and learned. Prepare for setbacks, obstacles, and do-overs, because humans learn by trial and error – there's no getting around it.

- Accept that you'll always be perfectly imperfect. Accept yourself just as you are, with your faults, mistakes, failures, regrets, anger, disappointment, embarrassments, and hurts. Realize that, just like every other human being, you have your own baggage, full of negatives you can correct, improve, or move beyond, if you want to. Accept that you also have talents, gifts, blessings, skills, accomplishments, and triumphs, just like any other human being. It's permissible to feel gratitude and joy over these positives. Life is confusing, glorious, complicated, and messy for everyone!

- Expand your concept of self. Many books on self-esteem and spirituality speak about the "true self" or "the higher self." Who you really are is a matter of belief, not provable as a fact. The test of a belief is not whether it's objectively true, but whether it serves a useful purpose. If so, it becomes subjectively true.

Let me tell you what I believe about who you really are. You are more than your possessions, relationships, looks, and roles. You are more than your struggles, failures, and triumphs. You are more than your body. These are all transitory. The real you, your true self, is eternal, ineffable, and transcendent. It is what remains after you take away everything that is merely acquired. What remains is beyond words because it is holy. It is made of the Infinite Consciousness that permeates and creates the universe and holds it together, differentiating every living entity, giving life and animation and endless variety. The life-giving force, the creative energy, universal knowledge – call it God, or what you will – is the essence of who you really are.

French priest and philosopher, Pierre Teilhard de Chardin (1881–1955) said: "We are not human beings having a spiritual experience. We are spiritual beings having a human experience." If you hold such a belief, then, inevitably, you cannot help but stand in awe of who you really are.

Tips for Improving Your Self-Esteem

Here are my favorite tips for improving self-esteem.

- **Look at yourself in the mirror.** Author, publisher, and speaker on holistic health, Louise L. Hay has, in her own words, dedicated her life's work to creating "a world where it is safe for people to love themselves." Read her bestseller on self-esteem called *You Can Heal Your Life*, and be inspired.[55] She has often taught "mirror-work": looking at yourself in a mirror and speaking to yourself with love.

  Stand before a mirror, look into your eyes, and say, "I love you with all my heart." When I have mentioned this to therapy groups, I am amazed at the terror on the faces of so many who can't imagine feeling such love for themselves. I've actually seen people burst into tears at the very suggestion! Mirror-work is amazingly powerful! Keep doing it until you can feel the love in your heart for that human being looking back at you.

- **Find your theme song.** Choose an uplifting song about love and life. Let it be your theme song. Frank Sinatra (1915–1998), for example, had "I Did It My Way." I think everyone should have their own theme song.

- **Surround yourself with happy, upbeat people.** Associate with people who come together out of common interests to share healing experiences, teach and support one another, or to share friendship and enjoyment. Find groups that fit your needs and match your values.

- **Keep a gratitude journal.** Take a few minutes each day or week to write about those things for which you feel grateful. Most of us complain far too much and take too little time to realize how richly our lives are blessed. Gratitude is a balm for the troubled soul.

- **Write a letter to your body.** Write a letter of reconciliation to your body. By loving your body, you achieve a measure of self-acceptance. Thank your body for all it does for you, without having to be reminded or told. Tell your body that you are willing to love it, respect it, honor it, and care for it with sufficient rest, sleep, activity, and nutrition. Promise you'll attend to your body's communication patterns. Hear your body saying "Thank you" in response.

- **Forgive.** Are you carrying around old resentments and guilt? Resentment is anger at others. Guilt is anger at self. Both are painful, yet both remind us that we have a sense of right and wrong, justice and injustice. Making peace with those who have harmed you doesn't mean you condone their actions. It means you are no longer willing to carry the burden of their wrongdoing. If you carry guilt, make amends to anyone you have harmed. If you can't make amends, then make atonement, such as volunteer work or community service, as homage to the person you have wronged. Talk about your guilt to a psychotherapist or member of the clergy. Let guilt be a stark way of fully realizing your values, and then resolve to live accordingly, a chastened but more authentic individual.

- **Give yourself credit.** Do you minimize your positives? I once had a client who said she had no self-esteem. I asked her to write 20 things she liked about herself. She couldn't think of *one*. I asked if she was a good parent. Yes. I asked if she was a good citizen who obeyed the law. Yes. I asked if she was a safe driver. Yes. Soon we had a list of 20 items. I asked her how it was that she had so much trouble coming up with these things. She said, "Oh I just take those things for granted. I didn't think they would count." Having good self-esteem means to give yourself credit for all you do well – skills, talents, and accomplishments – even those things you do every day. This is how to appreciate yourself. Now make *your* list of 20 things.

- **Develop spiritual practices.** Enrich your soul with practices such as reading, singing, prayer, or meditation. Decide the meanings of dreams, coincidences, intuitive messages, the divine, the mystical, pain and joy, peace and suffering, acceptance and confrontation, individuality and conformity. Socrates said, "The unexamined life is not worth living." How do you hear and follow your inner wisdom? What is your purpose? How do you rightly walk life's path?

- **Sense your boundaries.** Psychological boundaries allow you to define yourself physically and emotionally as separate from others. Self-esteem implies that you understand your boundaries. You can make your boundaries porous enough to allow emotional closeness and trust. At the same time, you can make your boundaries strong enough that you'll defend and protect yourself against those who might harm you or violate your dignity and privacy.

- **Validate yourself.** External validation comes in the form of compliments, praise, awards, and recognition. Internal validation comes from within. While you can appreciate and enjoy external validation, it's essential that you also validate yourself. Set meaningful goals and strive for realistic standards of accomplishment. Compare your results to your standards. If what you do isn't up to your standards, change your standards, or make corrections and improvements in your behavior. Give yourself credit for effort. Celebrate your accomplishments.

- **Reconcile with the past.** If you want to be authentically you, it is essential to reconcile with the past – your own mistakes, shortcomings, and suffering, as well as what others did to you or with you. To hold on to past pain is to live as a victim and an emotional hostage. To reconcile with the past is to live freely in the now moment, finding peace and joy as best you can. For more on this, see Chapter 19.

Note: If you are in an abusive relationship, please end that relationship or get help. Far too many people suffer at the hands of another. It is well-nigh impossible to feel competent and adequate if someone else is harming you. If someone else is blocking you from authenticity, consider whether it is worth it to maintain that relationship. You cannot reasonably expect to improve your self-esteem if you are in danger or facing any kind of harassment.

Additionally, if you have a history of unresolved abuse or trauma, it is unlikely you can reach emotional stability alone. Depression and anxiety can be debilitating, and are often related to significant emotional issues. Please seek the help of a psychotherapist and be prepared to invest in your well-being.

Self-Hypnosis: Increase Your Self-Esteem

This strategy was originally developed by L. Michael Hall.[56] In developing it, Hall identified three components of self-esteem:

- *Accepting* who you are, in spite of shortcomings.
- *Appreciating* what you do well.
- *Awe* for your potential; what you aspire to and what you can become.

This strategy guides you in accessing each of these three states, and then applying them to your self. *Self* means who you are as a unique individual living your own life experiences, with your own perceptions, emotions, values, and capabilities. This strategy layers positive thoughts about your self for a multiplying effect that creates a state of self-empowerment. Then you can amplify the state and mentally rehearse applying it in contexts where you want a more complete sense of self-esteem and self-valuing. Note that this strategy anchors three individual states (acceptance, appreciation, and awe), and then combines them for a really intense state of self-esteem. Here are the steps:

1. Induce and deepen trance with any method of your choosing.

2. Access and anchor, one at a time, a resourceful state of acceptance, appreciation, and awe. Access each state by remembering a situation in which you experienced that state. Choose a reminder word – a verbal cue for each of the three states – that will help you to access the state again.

   - **Acceptance:** Remember a situation in which you felt acceptance of something true about yourself, that you were not aware of until that moment. Perhaps someone paid you a compliment on a personal quality or acknowledged one of your skills, bringing it to your attention for the first time. Remember finding it true and accepting it. Be there now. See what you saw. Hear what you heard. Feel the state of acceptance. Choose a cue-word for that state. Return your thoughts to the here and now.

   - **Appreciation:** Think of something you do well, which you really appreciate as one of your skills or talents, or perhaps a positive achievement. Feel the glow of appreciation. Anchor that feeling with a cue-word.

- **Awe:** Think of your potential – all the aspirations that await your fulfillment. Realize the wonder of being alive to witness the beauty and complexity of the world. What excites you, intrigues you, and rivets your attention because it is so awesome? Let examples from your personal experience play through your mind. Really get into the state of awe. Anchor that feeling with a cue-word.

3. Amplify each state and apply it to your concept of yourself. To do so, imagine stepping into a bubble that holds each state. As you do, mentally say (even shout!) your cue-word for that state. Let the state permeate your being, radiating from you and around you as light and sound (maybe music). Immerse yourself in the feelings and bring those feelings to bear on being you.

   - Imagine moving into the bubble that holds your state of *acceptance*. Re-access the feelings of self-acceptance. Say your cue-word for this state. Let the state permeate your being, shining out from you and around you, with light, energy, and glorious sounds. Amplify the state by making it more intense – brighter, bigger, more colorful, or more pleasing in some way. Say, "I accept myself and all that I am, just as I am in this moment."

   - Imagine moving into the bubble that holds your state of *appreciation*. Re-access the feelings of appreciation. Say your cue-word for this state. Let the state permeate your being, shining out from you and around you, with light, energy, and glorious sounds. Amplify the state by making it more intense – brighter, bigger, more colorful, or more pleasing in some way. Say, "I appreciate myself!"

   - Imagine moving into the bubble that holds your state of *awe*. Re-access the feelings of awe. Say your cue-word for this state. Let the state permeate your being, shining out from you and around you, with light, energy, and glorious sounds. Amplify the state by making it more intense – brighter, bigger, more colorful, or more pleasing in some way. Say, "I stand in absolute awe of my life, my being, and my self."

- Combine these three states. Imagine all three bubbles merging and combining into one state of self-esteeming acceptance, appreciation, and awe. Step into this state. See the colors, light, and energy. Hear the sounds. Feel the emotions. Say, "I accept myself. I appreciate myself. I hold myself in awe." Understand that you can apply this state in future contexts and situations where it will be useful.

4. Mental rehearsal: Think of a specific context where these resources would be useful to you. This would be a context in which you previously felt negativity for yourself. Imagine yourself in that type of situation in the future, where you now access a state of resourceful self-esteem. Imagine you are there now. See what you would see. Hear what you would hear. Let your state of acceptance, appreciation, and awe for yourself transform your response to that situation. Practice this step until it feels comfortable.

5. Return your thoughts to the here and now. Imagine looking into your future, visualizing and anticipating how your life will be different with this new state of self-esteem. Think of resourceful responses you'll make to situations that were once challenging. Resolve to continue feeling and affirming self-acceptance, self-appreciation, and awe for your life and all its potential. Intuitively grasp additional changes in your actions and thinking that will automatically occur as your self-esteem continues to improve.

6. Return your thoughts to the here and now. Reorient and open your eyes.

As your self-esteem improves, you'll notice many changes taking place in your thinking and behaviors. Here are a few possibilities:

- You are less likely to engage in negative self-talk.

- You stop bemoaning lost opportunities and berating yourself for past mistakes.

- You stop comparing yourself unfairly to others.

- You worry less over the possibility that others may judge you and find fault with you.

- You learn to speak up for yourself appropriately.

- You establish boundaries to the extent that you comfortably say no to situations that put you at a disadvantage.

- You choose relationships in which you are treated with equality and respect.

- You stop second-guessing yourself; you are more willing to trust your intuition and impressions.

Self-Hypnosis: Change a Limiting Belief about Yourself

Beliefs guide our choices and decisions, express our values, and shape our lives. We act on beliefs without questioning their validity. In NLP, the ultimate test of a belief is not whether it's true but, instead, how well it serves us. Low self-esteem is based on a limiting belief about self. Limiting beliefs hold us back from reaching our potentials, making us feel discouraged and depressed. Listen to your negative self-talk and you'll occasionally hear beliefs that damage self-esteem. Here are typical examples:

- I'm not good enough ("for what" is usually not specified, so the implication is "for anything").

- I'll never have what I truly want (i.e., love, money, recognition, achievement, etc.).

- I'm not as ... (smart, talented, pretty, rich, etc.) as other people are (and the implication is "therefore I am inferior").

- There's not enough ... (love, money, good men, good women, jobs, etc.) to go around and the implication is "I'll never get mine." (This is the belief in scarcity.)

- No one will ever ... (want, love, like, understand, hire, appreciate, etc.) me.

- I will never overcome my past … (hurts, failures, regrets, mistakes, etc.).

Most limiting beliefs don't make logical sense. They just *feel* true and therefore compelling. Does one or more of these limiting beliefs sound familiar? If so, you'll now learn a strategy for overcoming limiting beliefs. This self-hypnosis session is an adaption of the NLP Walking Belief Change Pattern developed by NLP trainer Robert Dilts.[57] It involves discarding a limiting belief and replacing it with an empowering belief.

First, choose a limiting belief to discard. Then choose an empowering replacement belief. For example, if your limiting belief is "I'm not good enough …" then a suitable replacement could be, "I'm okay just as I am." Check your replacement for "fit." Does it feel right? Would having it present any consequences? If so, keep working with it until it feels right and fits in well with your values, goals, other beliefs, responsibilities, and obligations. With a statement of each belief (a limiting belief and an empowering replacement belief), you are ready to begin.

In this visualization, imagine walking a path of belief change. You'll see signposts along the way, marking each step in the process as you transition from an old, limiting belief to a new, empowering belief. Here are the steps:

1. Induce and deepen trance with any method of your choosing.

2. Visualize walking on a path through a pleasant natural setting. At intervals on the path, you'll see signposts. You'll stop and read each one.

3. **Signpost 1: Your Old Belief**. Stop walking. Mentally state the limiting belief. Listen to the internal voice. Focus on the feelings the belief engenders. What memories come to mind? How has holding on to this belief harmed you or blocked you? Give yourself permission to release this belief. Continue walking on the path.

4. **Signpost 2: Uncertainty and Doubt**. Stop walking. Feel uncertainty and doubt about that old belief. Think of reasons why it may be true. Think of reasons why it may be false. Listen to both sides of

the debate. Notice feelings on each side. You could choose one or the other. Begin to doubt this old belief. Continue walking on the path.

5. **Signpost 3: Museum of Old Beliefs**. Now you see a building. It is your Museum of Old Beliefs. This building contains all the out-dated beliefs of your past. Go inside and look around. See the beliefs on display. What do you see? Notice how it feels to see old beliefs that are no longer true. Look! There's an empty display case, set aside for your old, limiting belief. Place your old belief in this display. Exit the museum, leaving your old belief behind in the display. Take a deep breath and feel the relief! Continue walking on the path.

6. **Signpost 4: Your Preferred Belief**. Stop here. What is your new replacement belief? Say it to yourself. Do you like it? How would it be to have this belief? What changes would occur for you, physically, mentally, emotionally, and spiritually? Continue walking on the path.

7. **Signpost 5: Open to Believing**. Stop here. State your new belief again. Let your mind open up to this new belief and accept it. Look forward to having it. Continue walking on the path.

8. **Signpost 6: Your Sacred Beliefs**. Stop here. Look around. You've come to a holy place. As you step into this place, you realize it holds a record of your most highly prized beliefs. Review this record, reciting some of your sacred beliefs to yourself. Feel the sensations of commitment and assurance as you review these beliefs. These you know are true. Insert your replacement belief in the record, among your sacred beliefs. Feel the same commitment and assurance about your new belief. Say it in your mind, with the same voice and tonality that you use for your other sacred beliefs. Accept it as true. Exit the holy place of your sacred beliefs. Continue walking on the path.

9. **Signpost 7: Your Future is Ahead.** Stop here. You see now that this path leads to the future. Look backward for a moment. Appreciate that you've replaced that old limiting belief with a new, empowering belief. Look toward your future. What will be different about you from now on?

10. Mental rehearsal: Visualize what you'll be doing, thinking, and feeling differently, now that you love and accept yourself. Make these images as vivid as you can. Consider what will be different in terms

of your relationships, your decisions, your work and play, your health habits, and your communication patterns. Remember, you are programming change at the unconscious level.

11. Return your thoughts to the present. State your new belief now as an affirmation that will stay with you. Reorient.

Repeat your new belief often as an affirmation, so that it will settle into the fabric of your daily thoughts. You can use the pattern above for any limiting belief.

Self-Hypnosis: See Yourself through the Eyes of Love

Do others love you more than you love yourself? If so, this section is for you. For this self-hypnosis process, identify someone who really loves you. It could be a friend or family member. If you can't identify a friend or family member, choose a spiritual entity, such as a holy person, guardian angel, or patron saint. If you choose someone who is no longer in your life, make sure this is a person for whom you retain warm feelings.

Would you like to love yourself as much as this person loves you? You can. This self-hypnosis process is adapted from the NLP Loving Yourself Pattern developed by NLP trainers Tim Hallbom and Suzy Smith.[58] It teaches you to love yourself by temporarily shifting your perception to that of another person. Here are the steps:

1. Induce and deepen trance with any method of your choosing.

2. Visualize sitting comfortably, alone in a familiar setting, doing something you enjoy. While sitting there, think about this person who loves you and cares about you. Think about the ways in which this person conveys loving you. What does he love about you? Enjoy knowing how much this person loves you.

3. As your visualization continues, imagine this person is nearby, watching you, even though you don't know it. He is looking at you with love. Pretend that you leave your own body and step into his body. See yourself through his eyes, with his heart and his mind. You

now see yourself while feeling love, compassion, and understanding for yourself. Feel his love for you. Realize what he appreciates about you. Wouldn't you like to feel this way about yourself?

4. Return to your own body, bringing those loving feelings. Give all those feelings to yourself. Fully receive this love from another and, now, from yourself as well. Let your mind generate new insights and discoveries. Discover new information that enriches your sense of self. Say to yourself, "I am loved and lovable." Realize that this other person is still looking at you. Feel all the love he is sending. Let it soak you with good feelings.

5. Return to the here and now, bringing those loving, lovable feelings with you. Have those feelings right now. Project them into the future and anticipate having them more each day. Say to yourself, "I am loved and lovable," letting it become a daily affirmation.

6. Mental rehearsal: Think about a type of situation in which it has typically been difficult to be good to yourself. Imagine that type of situation occurring in the future. Be there now, fully loving yourself and being good to yourself. Notice what else changes. What if you took these loving feelings for yourself into future endeavors and relationships? Imagine moving into each day supporting yourself, taking care of yourself, giving yourself reassurances and encouragement, believing in yourself, forgiving your mistakes, and doing your best.

7. Return your thoughts to the here and now. Reorient and open your eyes.

The Meaning of Self-Esteem

On the desk in my office, I keep a chunk of rock that fits nicely in the palm of my hand. The rock is plain-looking, black and gray, with a craggy surface. I often use it as a metaphor about self-esteem. When a client tells me about low self-esteem, I take the rock and hold it in my hand. "Perhaps you could compare yourself to this rock," I say. "It's not much to look at. Nothing remarkable. Just an old rock...that is, until you look at it rightly."

At that point, I turn the rock over, to show that the rock is really a chunk of a geode. The interior reveals sparkling quartz and amethyst. Then I continue speaking. "At the core of this plain-looking rock, we see something beautiful and valuable. People are the same way. We have shortcomings, failures, and faults that render us imperfect. Nevertheless, at our core, we are all human beings. Somewhere in the course of becoming civilized, humans decided that even the worst and lowest among us should be treated with a basic fairness and dignity. That's because, we believe, at the core of each human being, there is something of value and worth that should not be violated but held sacred. The world's religions teach this message."

Positive self-esteem isn't based on being perfect or on comparing yourself to others. It's realizing that to be fully human is to struggle with ignorance, failings, and imperfections and love ourselves anyway. No one gets through life without being mistreated and insulted. No one gets through life without feeling guilty, ashamed, and inadequate at some point. No one gets through life without harming another. Nevertheless, we each have an opportunity (some would say a responsibility) to discover and reveal the unique gifts that we possess, to answer a calling to develop our strengths and talents, and to revel in the glory of living, loving, and learning as best we can. To live fully and authentically is to recognize your shortcomings and inadequacies and love yourself anyway. It is to acknowledge that life is often painful and unfair, and appreciate it anyway.

It's understandable if parts of this chapter have evoked some poignant emotions. The need for love and acceptance is woven into our genes. We sometimes forget that the love we most want is the love that comes from within. Until you love *yourself*, all the love in the world will never fill the void. I hope that this chapter has helped you to embrace who you are and enjoy what makes you a unique and precious child of the universe.

CHAPTER 16

Manage Your Emotions for Equanimity and Resilience

Do you remember, when you were a child, opening, for the first time, a brand new green and yellow box of Crayola® Crayons? Do you remember the waxy smell as you looked into the box and sensed a world of artistic possibilities in that rainbow of colored crayons? Like crayons in a box, our emotions color our lives. Even though we like some emotions and dislike others, it takes all the colors of our emotions to make our personalities complete. Every emotion has a purpose. Every emotion is appropriate in some context.

The problem arises when we fall into emotional patterns that are inappropriate for a particular circumstance. In the wrong context, emotions do more harm than good. Inappropriate emotions usually surface under conditions that we regard as difficult, challenging, or stressful. Sometimes we become so skilled at accessing these inappropriate emotions that we generalize them to a number of contexts. Our neurological structures adapt to repetition. So we reach the point where we consistently produce such emotions more quickly, frequently, and in a wider variety of circumstances.

If your emotions seem crippling, or could result in harm to yourself or others, or if you are in an abusive relationship, please get help. Many people approach therapy with the idea: "What good will it to do to talk about something I can't solve?" Well, most lay people aren't familiar with the newer therapies. With more recent approaches, such as NLP, it's possible, in a short time, to learn to release anxiety and panic, achieve deep relaxation, gain insights, and break the patterns of depression. A good therapist can help you out of the quagmire and develop a plan for change based on small, incremental steps – with ideas you probably hadn't thought about before. She can help you understand both the physiological and psychological aspects of your problem, and make referrals to community groups, clinics, alternative medicine practitioners, and physicians who specialize in your particular issue.

This chapter does not offer mental health therapy. It does provide strategies for working through difficult emotions and changing habitual emotional responses. The methods in this chapter are not analytical; they don't get at "why." They are solution-oriented; they get at "how" to produce the solution, so that you experience problematic emotions less and less, replacing them with more resourceful states.

Tips for Stress Management: Improve Your Coping Skills

Stress is a mind–body reaction to events that we perceive as threatening, harmful, or upsetting. We can all thrive on a moderate degree of stress, which can challenge us, test our coping skills, and push us out of our comfort zones. Overwhelming stress, however, can result in physical, mental, and emotional discomfort and illness. Stress begins when we experience or think about any emotionally dramatic life event. The event may be real or imagined, remembered from the past, happening right now, or anticipated in the future.

As the event registers, the limbic brain (the part of the brain that registers emotions) is activated and sends a cascade of neurochemical messenger molecules throughout the body to activate the autonomic nervous system, resulting in physical arousal. The neuro-endocrine system pours out adrenaline, resulting in a faster heartbeat and increased blood pressure. Digestion slows down to divert energy to the heart and brain. The pupils widen. The senses are more keen and alert. Muscles tense, ready for action. This is the flight-or-fight response. This response is useful, and sometimes life-saving, for those moments when we need a quick, short-term physical reaction – such as jumping out of the way of a speeding car.

While this fight-or-flight reaction is useful in some situations, it is not so helpful in response to ongoing pressures such as meeting work deadlines, managing a busy household, facing financial worries, coping with a daily commute, and confronting a constant overload of information, requirements, and responsibilities. The autonomic nervous system attempts to accommodate by maintaining a low and constant level of arousal, in which equanimity becomes elusive and difficult to achieve. At the end of the day, exhaustion sets in. The next day brings more of the same.

We can all weather occasional bouts of stress with no ill effects. However, when stress seems intense and/or unrelenting for days on end, then stress-related illness will often follow. Doctors now tell us that 80 percent of all illnesses have their origins in stress. Under emotional upheaval, people make fewer healthy decisions, judgment is impaired, the immune system is weakened, sleep patterns are disturbed, and fatigue sets in.

There are basically two ways to cope with stress. One is palliative and the other is instrumental. A palliative response seeks relief. An instrumental response seeks to change the situation. Palliative responses are the only course of action when the situation cannot be changed. The instrumental response is useful when taking action is an option; where it's possible to negotiate, object, reorganize, fight back, refuse, or leave. Either response can bring rewards or consequences. Sometimes a palliative response is the choice for people who feel too fearful to confront a difficult situation. They don't want up to upset the boat. Sometimes an instrumental response can result in a mistake or in unintended consequences. Nevertheless, doing something may seem better than doing nothing. Here are a few of my favorite stress management recommendations, which incorporate both types of response.[59]

Practice the Three P's. Whenever I have worked with clients who feel chronically anxious, worried, and distressed, I find that they often lack one of the three essential elements of effective coping. These three elements – people, purpose, and peace – can provide the foundation for the values and decisions that guide our daily actions.

- **People:** I believe it is essential for each of us to develop and maintain a safety net of loving, caring relationships with friends and family. We are, after all, social beings. Studies show that supportive relationships help people to more effectively weather stress, cope with loss, maintain better health, and recover faster from illness and surgery.

- **Purpose:** Without a sense of purpose, life seems directionless. Purpose is something to live for. It gives life a direction and shapes identity, values, and beliefs. An overriding sense of purpose gives meaning to life and might even sustain you in the face of tragedy. Purpose gives people the strength to go on living and planning for tomorrow.

- **Peace:** I believe it is necessary for everyone to have a spiritual practice and a system of faith that helps make sense of life. Cultivating a sense of inner peace will give you an emotional refuge in the face of chaos.

Maintain good healthcare practices. If you take care of yourself physically, you'll be less susceptible to stress-related illnesses. Here are the six best things you can do for your health:

1. Get regular medical checkups.
2. Don't smoke.
3. Get adequate and balanced nutrition.
4. Choose a safe exercise plan and follow it consistently.
5. Achieve and maintain a healthy weight.
6. Get seven to eight hours of sleep each night.

Develop an abundance mentality. Maintain an optimistic belief that your needs and desires can be satisfied. The abundance mentality is the belief that there is enough love, wealth, and happiness to go around and you can have your share, as well as feel happy for those who have theirs. With an abundance mentality, you count your blessings and feel gratitude for them, even in the midst of loss. Your attitude is that the glass is half full, not half empty. You approach challenges with optimism and faith in your ability to do your best.

Acquire a willingness to go to Plan B. If what you're doing isn't working, maybe it's time to consider a change of course. While having goals, a sense of purpose, and a plan are important to success, sometimes the unexpected can dramatically alter your life direction. You can sink into hopelessness and despair or you can regroup and go to Plan B. People who choose Plan B rebuild their lives after a loss or setback.

Make a realistic assessment of what you can control. Consider the Serenity Prayer by Reinhold Niebuhr, adopted for use by Alcoholics Anonymous: "God grant me the serenity to accept the things I cannot change, the courage to change the things I can, and the wisdom to know the difference." How often do you wallow in anger and anxiety and worry over something you cannot change? How often do you procrastinate and avoid making the changes that you can? It is often less stressful to surrender to the acknowledgement of what is beyond your personal control and direct your energies toward what is realistically possible.

Stop asking "Why?" and start asking "How?" When faced with a problem, many people say, "I have to know *why*." They believe that if they know why, then they will automatically find a solution. Most human problems have more than one cause. To assign the reason to a single cause is often overly simplistic. Knowing why a problem exists doesn't always lead to the solution. You won't get to the solution until you ask, "How can I solve this problem?"

Create a healthy relationship with the past, present, and future. Your mental relationship with time can be a factor in how well you cope with stress. People with a dysfunctional relationship with the past dwell on the hurts, disappointments, and mistakes of the past, and bring negative emotions into the present. They remain stuck in outdated fears, guilt, and resentments. People with a dysfunctional relationship with the future worry about the future, expect the worst, and bring negative emotions into the present, without even knowing what will come to pass. They rob themselves of any satisfaction with the present.

Holding on to the hurts of the past and seeing the future as dark and bleak is a perfect formula for depression. Conversely, a healthy relationship with the past, present, and future entails the ability to detach from negative events of the past, cherish the memories of good times and pleasure, make plans for the future based on reasonably optimistic expectations of success, and live fully in the present with a clear sense of identity, values, and purpose. A healthy relationship with the past, present, and future makes for a life well-lived.

Be willing to get help. No matter how smart or competent you are, you can't master every challenge alone. Recognize when you are in over your head and get some help. Studies show that people who participate in mutually supportive relationships with friends and family are healthier than those who don't. Also consider sources of professional help – counselors, life coaches, and therapists. If you enjoy reading, there seems to be an ample supply of self-help books for almost any difficulty. You can also find biographies of people who once faced difficulties and challenges that are similar to yours and who surmounted those obstacles and found inner strength. Reach out and find the help you need. When the student is ready, the teacher appears.

Manage time. The two biggest time management issues for most people are (1) too much to do in too little time and (2) procrastination. Too much to do results in feeling overwhelmed and fatigued. Procrastination leads to feeling guilty and frustrated. Here are some time management tips to get control over your schedule.

- Decide on your priorities. You can set your priorities for the year, the month, the week, and for today. These are the things you absolutely must accomplish within that time frame.

- Break large tasks into smaller chunks so that the chunks are easier to accomplish in a shorter time frame.

- Make a daily to-do list each morning as you plan your day. Highlight the priorities. Schedule time to work on priority items. Number the remaining items in order of importance and work through the list from the most important to least important items. What you don't accomplish today gets moved to tomorrow's list.

- Eliminate activities that waste your time and energies. Time wasters can include phone time, surfing the internet, computer games, moving clutter from place to place, searching for misplaced items, idle television watching, etc.

- Say "no" (tactfully) to responsibilities and requests from other people that do not support your priorities. Stop volunteering for every committee and worthy cause. Yes, others could use your skills and talents, but they can't reduce your stress, nor can they lessen your work load.

- Think of ways to save time. What can you delegate? What can you pay someone else to do? Is there a time-saving appliance that will help to simplify your work? Tell yourself that it's okay to take an occasional short cut – such as ordering carry-out instead of cooking a large meal for unexpected guests.

- You can conquer procrastination if you know what you are telling yourself. Identify the task on which you are procrastinating and ask yourself, "What is it about doing this task that causes me to keep putting it off?" Your answer will give you a clue as to the remedy. See Chapter 12 for more information.

Manage space. The two toughest two space management issues for most people are too many possessions and not enough space. Our possessions expand to fill the space we have, and often the space we have is overflowing, making for disorganization and clutter. We complain that we don't have enough room for all our household possessions and activities. Here are two tips:

- Implement storage solutions that store similar items in one place. Invest in shelving, storage boxes, file cabinets, and organization systems for pantries, laundry rooms, closets, and garages.

- Design the rooms of your home for multiple purposes. A study with a fold-out bed can double as a guest room. Set up a treadmill in your recreation room, so that you can watch television or listen to music and burn calories at the same time. A kitchen table can double as a desk or extra work space for hobbies.

Manage clutter. In our affluent, consumer-oriented society, we buy and receive things. We collect things. We acquire things. Things often lead to clutter. Clutter takes extra time because you have sort through it and work around it to find what you are looking for. Clutter looks messy and gives a feeling of chaos and discouragement. Here are a few clutter solutions:

- Make an appointment with yourself (and family members, as needed) to resolve a cluttered area in your home. Typical clutter areas are home offices, closets, drawers, garages, file cabinets, and basements. Put everything in a pile in the middle of the room. Sort the large pile into six smaller piles and take action on each one:

  1. What you no longer need – things to throw away. (Note: Shred confidential paperwork.)

  2. What you can give to someone you know.

  3. What you can donate to charity.

  4. What you can still use with a few updates, modifications, mending or repair.

  5. (Optional) Items you can resell – think yard sale or eBay®.

  6. What you'll keep as is. For these items, devise a storage system.

- Paperwork is usually the largest source of clutter. The solution to paperwork is a filing system.

There are plenty of good self-help "get organized" books on the market. I recommend is *It's All Too Much* by organizational guru, Peter Walsh.[60] You could also consider hiring a storage expert or organizing specialist to help turn your messiness into efficiency.

Things require time, energy, and space. When we own too many things, we spend excessive money to provide space for it all. Then we have to work more to earn more money to pay for the space. Things require maintenance, too – another expense. They often become obsolete before they wear out. You can simplify your life with fewer possessions.

Resolve unfinished business, be done with it, and move on. It takes wisdom to know when enough is enough. Do you hold on to old hurts and resentments? Do you keep trying to salvage that hurtful relationship? Do you make the same blunders over and over? Do you keep a closet full of out-of-date clothes that you don't even like because someday they may fit again? Do you store broken appliances because someday you might get them repaired – yet you never do? At some point, it's a good idea to clear up unfinished business and move on.

Practice risk management. Almost all worthwhile endeavors are fraught with the risk of danger, disappointment, and/or failure. Yet, if we don't take risks, we'd never accomplish anything of lasting value. We'd never pursue our dreams. How do you get what you want and pursue your goals in the face of risk? In business, decision-makers use "risk management." It's a process of first assessing risks and then finding ways to mitigate them. Here is a way to do it. First, take off the rose-colored glasses and acknowledge that risks do exist. Then ask yourself these questions:

- If I pursue this course, what is the worst that can happen?

- If I don't pursue this course, what is the worst that can happen?

- What is the probability (high, medium, or low) of that happening?

- If it did happen, could I live with it?

- If it did happen, could I still continue toward my goal?

- If it did happen, could I recover sufficiently?

- Given that this risk is possible, then how could I best avoid or prevent this risk or mitigate its impact?

- Given my answers, am I prepared to move forward?

Make risk management a part of your planning. Establish your priorities and risk tolerances, exercise reasonable precautions, and forge ahead.

Find a middle ground between exaggerating problems and avoiding them. What you tell yourself about the severity of an event can often affect how you respond. Some people interpret every minor mishap as a disaster! Other people ignore problems and avoid conflict, hoping the problem will get better or go away by itself – yet they simmer in resentment, feeling powerless. The challenge is to distinguish between a minor mishap and a true catastrophe. When you face a challenge, rank the situation on a scale from one to ten, with ten being the worst you can imagine. Realize that most things that stress us are not at the level of a ten. Match your problem-solving skills, and your emotions, to the size of the problem.

Appreciate the rewards of positive self-talk. Negative self-talk stirs up negative emotions, placing stress on the body. What we tell ourselves often becomes a self-fulfilling prophecy. Think realistically positive thoughts and your mood might change for the better.

Get Past Anxiety-Producing Thoughts and Negative Inner Dialog

Anxiety, anger, resentment, guilt, excessive worry, and self-loathing are often expressed and/or triggered by an intrusive, negative, inner voice. Some people call it the "inner critic" or the "thought demon." Most people have no idea how to stop this critical, nagging inner voice. Trying to ignore it or "turn it off" just doesn't work!

NLP trainer Nick Kemp, who manages Provocative Change Works™ in Leeds, England, has found that this negative inner voice is often instantly recognizable, with a particular tonality and, typically, a fast pace. He has developed a simple and reliable method for stopping that inner voice.[61]

1. First, examine your feelings to make certain you feel congruent about eliminating this voice. Check to discover any positive intention in the message that you would want to acknowledge and honor.

2. Close your eyes and bring up the negative inner voice. Hear what it usually says. If you aren't sure of the exact words, just make them up. Hear the tonality and pace. Be aware of the feelings that accompany the voice.

3. Internal voice tempo change: Say the words aloud, at the same pace and tonality. Say them again, but slow them down to one-third normal speed. Repeat, and show the words to one-half normal speed. Repeat, and hear the words one at a time, at an even slower speed, pausing longer before the last two words.

4. Test: Try to bring up the inner voice again and notice any changes. Usually it will be weaker, or will have disappeared altogether. Your feeling response will also be different and possibly non-existent.

Kemp also developed a visual variation on the internal voice tempo change:

- Visual variation: Visualize the words in a sentence in front of you, in your visual field. Note the color, font size, and style of the letters. Spread the words out, making wider spaces between them. Study the spaces between the words. Separate the letters of the words, making spaces between them. Study all the spaces between the words and letters. Keep spacing the words and letters out until they no longer make sense.

Kemp wrote: "In some instances I may then get the client to run both the auditory and the visual versions of this exercise at the same time. To date, I've used this with around 300 clients and in a single pass. No client has been able to get back their original sentence with the original response" (p. 3).

The two strategies above incorporate changes to the submodalities of internal representations. These strategies are based on an NLP maneuver called "pattern interruption." It follows the work of Erickson. He often told his patients to engage in their particular problem pattern, but to alter or interrupt one element of the pattern, causing it to extinguish itself. When you think of it, every time you apply a new strategy to a problem, you are interrupting the pattern somehow. Pattern interruptions change the auditory and visual submodalities of the way in which we perform a problem. Apply the method above to your negative inner voice and discover what happens. Below are more pattern interruptions:

- Change the location of the inner voice: Determine which side of your head the voice seems to come from (right or left). Move the voice around to the opposite side.

- Change the identity of the inner voice: Make it speak like Donald Duck or Mickey Mouse. Give it a foreign accent.

- Change the volume of the inner voice: Make the voice a muffled whisper, coming from far away, even in the next room. Say, "What? I can't hear you."

- Change the entire experience into a metaphor: See the words floating above your head in a pink thought balloon. Imagine that you reach up with a pin and pop the balloon and watch it burst into hundreds of tiny pieces and disintegrate.

When you get the voice to go away, mentally rehearse. Visualize a type of situation where you've typically heard the negative inner voice. Imagine being in that same type of situation but without the negative voice. In fact, notice the thoughts that automatically replace the negative inner voice.

Self-Hypnosis: Stress Management with NLP – Anchor a New Response

When it comes to coping with stressors, you have three choices. You can change the situation, remove yourself from the situation, or change your response to the situation. Given the extent to which stress is physically damaging, if you can't reasonably change the situation or remove yourself from it, then it behooves you to change your own response. By this, I mean that you change your emotions, thoughts, and actions so that you respond to the situation more resourcefully. Even if you are in the "right" and the situation is wrong or unfair, if your response is to succumb to stressful emotions, then it is not a useful response.

The question is this: If a particular situation has reliably triggered your unresourceful response, then how do you switch to a better response? The answer lies in an NLP strategy called *anchoring*, which allows you to consistently replace an unwanted emotion with another, more resourceful emotion. Here is a self-hypnosis strategy based on anchoring. Read the steps carefully before doing them in trance, to understand the underlying psychological mechanism. It's based on classical conditioning – the same method Pavlov used when he taught dogs to salivate to a bell. You'll condition a resourceful response to a trigger that once signaled difficult emotions.

Here are the steps:

1. Induce trance in any manner you choose.

2. Look objectively at your unwanted response in a typically problematic situation. Visualize this imagery in a dissociated manner, as though watching a movie of yourself. Notice exactly what triggers your response.

3. Visualizing that movie, ask yourself, "What resourceful state would I need to handle that situation more effectively?"

   Think carefully about the answer. When I ask that question, my clients usually say "calm" or "relaxed" because those states immediately spring to mind. Calm or relaxed might be ideal, but consider other options as well: patient, confident, curious, poised, forgiving, helpful, humble, detached, assertive, persistent, creative, or humorous are all potentially appropriate responses to difficult circumstances. Choose your resourceful state.

4. Bring your thoughts back to the here and now.

5. Identify an unrelated situation (a different context from the problematic one) in which you consistently and reliably demonstrate your resourceful state. Mentally access that state, in the appropriate context, visualizing it in an associated manner. Imagine that you are there, "in person" so to speak. Have the thoughts and feelings typical of that state.

6. Pair your resourceful state with a distinct cue that you can control (a word, or a tactile sensation, such as squeezing two fingers together).

7. Repeat Steps 3 and 4 three to five times to condition the response.

8. Return your thoughts to the here and now.

9. Visualize that you are in the problematic situation. This time, instead of watching a movie, you are there, fully associated. At the moment

that you experience the trigger, apply your conditioned cue. Instantly access a resourceful state, thinking quality thoughts, feeling appropriate emotions. Play out the scenario. Imagine what you are doing, saying, thinking, and feeling.

10. Repeat Step 9 three to five times, tweaking your imagined response for small improvements.

11. Bring your thoughts back to the here and now.

12. Mental rehearsal: Imagine the next time you encounter the type of situation that was problematic for you. Visualize responding to that situation in this new way with a much more resourceful response.

13. Return your thoughts to the here and now. Reorient and open your eyes.

Self-Hypnosis: Get Unstuck with the NLP Drop Down and Through Pattern

If you get stuck in persistent, negative emotions, such as worry, depression, or anxiety, this next self-hypnosis strategy is for you. Drop Down and Through is a meta-stating pattern, meaning that it is an exploration of the emotions we have about our emotions.[62] The idea here is that pervasive emotions are often difficult to dismiss because they are "layered" in meanings.

Think of layered emotions as a weed. If you just pull out the stem, the weed *seems* to go away. However, the roots are still there, under the soil. Soon the weed grows back. Until you get to the root, you won't eradicate the weed. The Drop Down and Through strategy is a highly contemplative method for getting to the root of a negative emotion and eradicating it. Here are the steps:

1. Induce trance with any method of your choosing.

2. Access the persistent emotion that has been difficult for you. Bring up the thoughts and feelings that most commonly characterize the emotional state.

3. Inhale. As you slowly exhale, imagine that you drop down and through the emotion, to a deeper level. Discover the meanings, images, thoughts, memories, and emotions that lie beneath. Notice what is here to learn. You will probably have insights and make connections of which you were not previously aware.

4. Repeat Step 3 a few more times (usually three to five times will suffice), until you reach a layer of nothing. This layer will be like a void, a darkness, or a shadow. There will be no feeling.

5. Drop down through the void to one more level. This state will be positive, pleasant, and peaceful. Anchor this state with a word or a touch.

6. Imagine that you are taking the anchored feeling back up through the layers, one at a time, transforming all the meanings at each level. Notice that the feelings and images at each layer change also. Advance slowly, transforming each layer until you get all the way back to the original emotional state.

7. Notice how the original state has changed.

8. Mental rehearsal: Imagine going through your day with this change in place. Imagine new feelings, thoughts, and behaviors. Imagine encountering a type of situation that previously has been challenging with this new state. Imagine what you'll be doing that will indicate an improvement has taken place.

9. Bring your thoughts back to the here and now. Reorient and open your eyes.

In completing this self-hypnosis session, you might want to journal about your insights and discoveries, or discuss them with a close friend, to process them.

Self-Hypnosis: Banish Fear and Anxiety with a Protective Shield

The archetypal image of a protective shield is pervasive in mythology. A protective shield is a metaphor for safety and the courage to approach difficult situations with equanimity. This self-hypnosis session combines relaxation with metaphoric imagery to suggest a psychological shield that protects you from negativity or unwanted influences. It can also alleviate unwarranted fear and anxiety and increase confidence. Here are the steps:

1. Induce trance with any method of your choice. Deepen your trance with progressive relaxation.

2. Affirmation: Give yourself the suggestions: I feel relaxed, peaceful, and calm. I feel safe and secure.

3. Releasing imagery: Imagine you are floating in a pool of emerald green water, looking up at a clear blue sky. You float serenely. All unwanted patterns of tension, fear, or anxiety are draining away, dissolving in the clear, cool water. All unnecessary thoughts of fear, worry, or anxiety are draining out of your mind, dissolving in the water. Natural beauty surrounds you: trees, flowers, and green grass. The air is fresh and sweet. Birds are singing. Frogs are chirping. You feel carefree, safe and secure, peaceful and calm. All is well.

4. Metaphoric imagery: Imagine a ray of sunlight, a beam of energy, shining down on you, narrowing, and coming to a point at your solar plexus. The energy is pure, benevolent, and soothing. It is a gift from the divine source. The energy moves into your body, bringing deeper relaxation, yet strengthening your neurological structures with equanimity and fortitude.

    The light circulates throughout your body, flowing through organs and muscles, streaming into arms and legs, healing the emotional residue of past events. It moves into your brain, activating resourceful thinking and new understandings and perceptions. It surges through your neurological structures, reorganizing faulty connections and pathways. It embeds itself in neuropeptides, moving into cellular receptors. It bathes every cell, organ, muscle, nerve, and tissue in compassionate bliss. Your unconscious is creating new associations.

    The light glows in your body, shining out through your skin, extending an arm's length beyond your body. The light surrounds you, as an energy field, enveloping you in contentment. The light now transforms its mission into one of protection.

The outer perimeter of the light forms a semi-permeable membrane that automatically filters out and deflects negativity, allowing only positive energies to flow in. You are surrounded by this invisible, protective shield – a bubble of light. Negativity bounces off the outer edges. When others seem unkind, you can see them and hear what they say, but their negativity bounces off your shield while you feel safe, in the bubble, maintaining equanimity and resilience. Imagine the sound of negativity bouncing off your shield – Clunk!

5. Return your thoughts to the –here and now. How would it be to go through your daily activities feeling protected and safe within your shield?

6. Mental rehearsal: Visualize a type of situation that has been anxiety-provoking. Imagine that you now encounter that situation while surrounded by your protective shield. Imagine how resourceful you feel when you notice negativity bouncing off the outer perimeter of your shield, "Clunk! Clunk! Clunk!" Imagine what you'll think, say, and do now that you have this degree of calm control, this clarity of thought, and this much resilience.

7. Return your thoughts to the –here and now. Reorient and open your eyes.

With this method, you can feel un-insultable. I have found it to be extremely helpful for children who get taunted in the playground and for adults who have to endure rudeness in the workplace. It is also useful for teachers who encounter defiant students, and performers and speakers who must cope with difficult audiences. The protective shield metaphor can stay with you, to help you feel calm and focused while you take appropriate action in response to a difficult situation.

Self-Hypnosis: Resolve Internal Conflict with the NLP Visual Integration Pattern

In Chapter 2, I mentioned that hypnosis doesn't always work due to internal conflict, which can often keep us stuck in indecision and anxiety. The NLP Visual Integration Pattern below was adapted from Richard

Bandler as a way to resolve such conflict creatively.[63] It's a reframing method, meaning that it changes the cognitive framework in which you typically think about a conflict.

We generally characterize an internal conflict as competing objectives. Internal conflict feels like a tug-of-war between two sub-personalities or "parts" of the self. One part of your mind wants one thing, and another part wants something else. Sometimes we say, "Intellectually I know I should do this, but my feelings tell me to do something else." We also experience an inner conflict when we feel guilty or angry with ourselves for a bad habit, but we feel compelled, nevertheless, to continue the habit.

With this method, you'll work with two internal parts. You'll represent each part as an image that you'll assign to either your left hand or right hand. You'll discover the positive intentions that drive each part. Then you'll help the parts "negotiate" a solution that satisfies both intentions. To negotiate between the parts, chunk up the positive intentions to notice what they have in common. Instead of "either–or" the solution becomes "both–and."

A note about positive intentions: it's an NLP principle that problem-atic behaviors are supported by underlying positive intentions of which we are often not conscious. Intentions reveal the hidden dynamics of unwanted behaviors and emotions. Sometimes the positive intention is initially expressed as a *hurtful* intention: something like "to punish you," or "to make you ashamed." If you encounter a hurtful intention, then ask again, "What is the positive intention of *that* (i.e., to punish you, make you ashamed). Eventually you'll discover a positive intention.

Before you begin the self-hypnosis process below, distinguish the two sides of your conflict as follows: "One part of myself wants to ... and the other part wants to ..." We will call the two parts A and B. Now complete the steps.

1. Sit in a chair with your hands on your lap or on the arms of a chair, palms up. You can complete this self-hypnosis method with your eyes open or closed. Induce trance with any method you choose.

2. Visualize the two parts as small, three-dimensional images, holding one image in each hand. The images can be anything – pictures of yourself, symbolic objects, cartoon characters, and so on. Give each part a "voice" with which to speak to you through your thoughts. These images represent the two parts of the self that are in disagreement. At this point, they may not like each other very much.

3. Hold a dialog with each part, one at a time. Begin with part A. Visualize part A in your hand. Mentally ask it, "What is your positive intention?" Wait patiently and let the answer come into your mind intuitively. Don't force the answer. When you are aware of the positive intention, appreciate that this value or need has come to your attention. Thank Part A.

4. Repeat for Part B.

5. Understand that although both A and B hold positive intentions, they interfere with each other's ability to fully actualize those positive intentions. Notice, however, their common goal. What do they *both* want for you?

6. Transform each part to a miniature image of yourself. Imagine the two parts looking at each other, talking about their positive intentions, and discovering their common goals. Ask them to agree to combine and share their resources and energies to more fully achieve all their positive intentions in ways that are healthy, appropriate, and safe.

7. Imagine each image reaching out for the other in friendship.

8. Slowly bring your hands together, palm to palm, as the two parts negotiate and cooperate, sharing their energies and resources as partners. This integration normally evokes pleasant feelings. Assume creative changes are forming within your unconscious as it works out "both–and" solutions.

9. When your hands touch, the integration is complete. Hold your hands together for a while, contemplating your inner experience. New ideas, solutions, and feelings may be evident. If not, simply thank the two parts for participating. Ask them to continue their negotiations, outside of your awareness, to arrive at creative solutions and agreements that lead to resolution.

10. Place your palms against your heart as the parts return to your body. Anticipate that you'll notice indications that resolution is now in progress. Reorient.

If solutions aren't immediately evident, assign the problem to your unconscious. Let it germinate there for a while. You might be delighted by changes that eventually occur.

The Misguided Need for Control

The majority of clients I see who suffer from panic, worry, tension, and anxiety have one common problem. They all have an exaggerated need for control. I don't guess at this: they tell me, "I'm a control freak! I have to be in control. If I'm not in control, I'm not happy." When I ask, "In control of what?" they say "Everything!"

No wonder they feel anxious and worried. To be in control of *everything* is impossible. In trying to be in control of everything, they lose control of the only things they can control – their own thoughts, feelings, and behaviors. When I ask, "How much control do you have over feeling anxious and worried?" the answer is, "None whatsoever."

It's the same with addictions like smoking, drugs, and overeating. They are often "out-of-control" attempts at control over circumstances that seem otherwise uncontrollable. Those who smoke say that they smoke to get control over anxiety and stress, but how much control do they have over smoking and the subsequent health risks? People who consistently overeat often say they turn to food to get control over boredom or loneliness, but they end up with out-of-control eating and out-of-control weight gain. We all know about the out-of-control behaviors of people who are desperate for their next drug fix.

When I ask people who smoke, take illegal drugs, or overeat what is so important about their habits, they tell me that the habit calms down their difficult emotions – gives them a sense of control – so they can handle daily life. Paradoxically, daily life eventually gets harder to handle with unwanted habits and addictions. When I ask, "And how much control do you have over smoking (or taking drugs or overeating)?" the answer is always the same: "None whatsoever."

The simple fact of life is that most things are not under our control. We really can't do much about the weather, the economy, crime rates, traffic, noise, pollution, the cost of living, large-scale tragedies, what other people do, and those two certainties – taxes and death. The excessive need for control is a fear-based, ego-based illusion.

It is fear-based because it activated by the fear of things that could go wrong. Often it is the desire to control things that are uncontrollable, unpredictable, and improbable. It is the fear of "What if …" What if the plane crashes? What if other people do things I don't like? What if something terrible happens to my loved ones? What if I get sick? What if I die? What if I make a fool of myself? A coward dies a thousand deaths and a neurotic endures a thousand tragedies. These are good ways to scare yourself, but not good ways to feel safe, confident, competent, or calm. What if you stop worrying and think rationally for a change? You can never anticipate every bad thing that could possibly happen, so why waste your energy?

It is ego-based because it presumes that you should be in charge of events, and other people and the world should behave according to your wishes. This is not likely to happen. Since you aren't in charge, you won't be bothered with having to come up with solutions and answers.

Instead of the futile task of trying to take control, why not take responsibility? Response-ability is the ability to respond to whatever happens, in a way that is consistent with your life purpose, beliefs, and values. If you really believe that good health is an essential part of a fulfilled life, then why are you smoking or drugging or overeating? Take responsibility for your health and throw away the cigarettes, get clean, get on a good nutritional plan, and start exercising. If you value serenity and inner peace, then take responsibility for your thinking and stop scaring yourself. Meditate, read inspirational books, journal, pray.

Don't know how to relax? A good therapist can teach you. Don't know your purpose in life? Find one. Choose it or let it choose you. Purpose gives life meaning and keeps you going, despite setbacks. It gives you determination and motivation, even when the odds are against you. When you really get honest about what matters, decisions become easier. It's not a matter of what you can control, but what serves your purpose, supports your values, and fulfills your passions.

Responsibility means doing things you don't necessarily like or enjoy because you are willing to do whatever it takes (in accordance with your morals, ethics, and values) to accomplish the outcomes you want. Doing whatever it takes might mean making big changes in your lifestyle, your health practices, your communication skills, and your thinking patterns. It might mean taking a good long look at your shortcomings and facing up to the fact that you are not yet an expert on the art of living, and you'd do well to find reputable teachers, mentors, and role models.

It helps to remember that the ultimate demonstration of control is the ability to release the need for control.

CHAPTER 17

Pain Management and Relief

Pain management is one the most frequent applications of hypnosis. Whether you contend with chronic or acute pain, hypnosis can provide considerable relief.

Acute pain serves a purpose. It is a signal from the body indicating an injury or malfunction. It's a message to remedy the situation. Once you've done what pain has signaled you to do, acute pain gradually decreases and eventually goes away. However, there is another kind of pain that lingers on, even when you've done everything possible. Chronic pain is pain that has outlived its usefulness. Self-hypnosis can help with acute pain and is especially beneficial in managing chronic pain.

Pain affects the body and mind in three main ways:

1. Injury or illness alerts nerve endings throughout the body to send pain signals to the pain receptors in the brain. We feel the discomfort of pain.

2. Pain receptors in the brain activate the amygdala – the brain's fear center – which in turn excites the sympathetic nervous system. Blood flow is restricted in the extremities and muscles tense throughout the body. Pain feels worse with this muscle tension and anxiety.

3. Attentional centers in the brain direct awareness toward the pain. Pain monopolizes attention, making it difficult to concentrate on anything else. Thus pain affects emotions and judgment.

Correspondingly, self-hypnosis can reduce pain in three ways.

1. Self-hypnosis facilitates visualization, drawing activity away from the pain receptors. Hypnosis is effective for pain management because it actually changes the brain's state. There is some speculation that

hypnosis actually "inhibits" the body's pain messages and the related brain activity.[64]

2. Self-hypnosis promotes muscle relaxation, calms anxiety, and reduces sympathetic nervous system activity.

3. Self-hypnosis directs attention away from pain, so that it becomes possible to ignore pain or to put it into the background of awareness.

Hypnosis and Pain

Hypnosis makes it possible to get conscious control over pain. A structure in the brain, called the periaqueductal gray (PAG), sets your pain threshold. The PAG is loaded with endorphins and opiate receptors modulated by emotion. Your perception of pain passes through this gateway and is strongly informed by emotions. The PAG isn't in the frontal cortex but the two are connected through neural pathways, making it possible to mentally modulate pain.[65]

Hypnosis can supplement and sometimes replace pain-relief medications. Hypnosis has been shown effective in mitigating pain from cancer,[66] burns,[67] and fibromyalgia.[68] An analysis of 18 studies of more than 900 people conducted at the Mount Sinai School of Medicine in New York found that hypnosis brought substantial pain relief to 75 percent of participants.[69] In fact, hypnosis was more effective than biofeedback, relaxation, cognitive-behavioral therapy, acupuncture, and morphine for both acute and chronic pain.

Self-hypnosis is useful not only for existing pain. It is also useful as a preparatory measure for anticipated pain, such as that associated with medical procedures. Let's say you are going for a medical exam in which you'll have blood drawn with a hypodermic needle. You can hypnotize yourself ahead of time to feel relaxed during the procedure, so fascinated by the objects in the examining room that you forget to notice the needle at all, hardly feeling the insertion.

There are dozens of hypnotic methods for reducing pain. The methods in this chapter are a mere sampling. For a comprehensive book on self-hypnosis for pain management, read *Hypnotize Yourself Out of Pain Now!*

by clinical psychologist and hypnotherapist Bruce Eimer.[70] You could also engage the services of a professional hypnotherapist to help develop imagery and suggestions for working with your particular type of pain.

I know about chronic pain on a personal level. I endured severe back and joint pain for many years. I was fortunate to find a holistic sports chiropractor who taught me how to recover through stretching and core-strength training. Today I am pain-free. My favorite affirmation is: "I move and rest in ease and comfort." Another is: "My comfort increases daily." I've found both of these to be helpful and, fortunately, prophetic.

Before we turn to self-hypnosis methods, bear in mind one caveat: hypnosis is not a substitute for proper medical treatment. If you have pain that requires medical attention, see your physician first.

Self-Hypnosis: Deep Relaxation

Begin with progressive relaxation as shown in Chapter 5. Deepen your relaxation, using additional induction methods shown in Chapter 5. Add, for example, the staircase induction. End your self-hypnosis session with a reorientation. Experiment to find the combination of methods that works best for you. Eimer recommended that, as you relax, you also make soothing suggestions to yourself, such as the following:

- My mind is quiet and still.

- My body is calm and relaxed.

- I am safe and at peace.

- Stress just drains away like water flowing out through a hole in bottom of a glass.

- I breathe in relaxation and breathe out tension and stress.

For additional pain reduction, select one or more of the methods in the remainder of this chapter and add it to your self-hypnosis deep relaxation session.

Self-Hypnosis: Imagery for Pain Reduction

Begin your self-hypnosis session with an induction and deepening method of your choice. Then, select imagery that represents an antidote, matching your subjective experience of pain. Use creativity. End with a reorientation. Here are a few examples:

- If your pain feels like the grip of a tight vise, imagine that part of your body in the vise. See the handle on the vise slowly turning counter-clockwise – opening the vise. See the "jaws" of the vice opening wide, releasing, and relieving the pain. See your capillaries and arteries and veins opening up so that the blood flows freely to the area.

- If your pain feels hot or burning, imagine that you go to your freezer. You fill up a pitcher with ice. You close the freezer and go to the sink. You turn on the tap, pouring cool, clear, fresh water into the pitcher. You hear the water running. You shut off the tap. You hear the tinkle of the ice floating in the water. Imagine now that you slowly and gently pour that ice water over the painful spot. See your skin changing its hue to indicate it is getting moist and cool. Imagine the coolness of the water penetrating beneath the skin and seeping deep into the muscles and tissues. Feel that spot getting cooler and much more comfortable.

- If the pain feels itchy or irritating, imagine a large bottle of lotion marked "soothing comfort." Make the bottle, and the lotion inside, a soothing color. Visualize pouring the lotion into the pain. The lotion is soft, moist, and gentle. The lotion spreads out over the painful area, bringing soothing relief. See the area soaking up the lotion and turning the color of the lotion. Imagine the lotion going down into the tissues and muscles, penetrating, soothing, cooling, and massaging the pain away.

- If the pain feels tight, mentally direct blood flow to the area. Visualize capillaries, veins, and arteries opening up and carrying an increased volume of blood to the area. Imagine the tissues getting warmer and receiving the blood flow. Feel the pulsations as more blood reaches the area. If you don't actually feel the pulsations, imagine that you do and your body will respond.

- For throbbing pain, imagine the blood flow in the veins and arteries pulsating in that area. Then, using the same method as above, direct the blood flow away from the site, to another part of your body. Concentrate your attention on a body area that is remote from the pain. Feel every sensation in that other, pain-free area. Visualize the blood flow to the pain-free area. Concentrate to the point that you can feel your pulse in that location. Imagine the pulse rate increasing as you mentally direct the blood flow to that location.

- If your pain feels like a tight knot, visualize the painful area as a piece of rope tangled up in knots. See the color and texture of the rope. Slowly watch the rope untangle as, one by one, the knots untie themselves, as you feel more and more comfortable. Imagine how the rope looks as the knots disappear.

Here are a few generic pain management scripts, especially useful for pain that defies description.

- In *Imagery for Getting Well*,[71] author Deirdre D. Brigham offered a variety of images for pain relief. In one, she told readers to imagine that a large, indigo-blue silk scarf floats down from the sky. Imagine, she advised, that the scarf comes to rest in your hands. You fold it and place it over the painful area, allowing your body to absorb the scarf. The scarf wraps around the pain, trapping the pain in the fabric. Then, a corner of the scarf reappears, peeping out through a small pocket in your skin. You gently withdraw the scarf, pulling out all the pain, feeling comfort and relief. You drop the scarf into a nearby wastebasket and walk away.

- Visualize walking on a path through a forest on a warm, spring day. See the trees with new leaves; flowers in bloom. Birds are singing. You arrive at a clearing with soft grass. The path leads down through the grass to a beautiful pond. The water is a deep indigo-blue. Slip into the cool, soothing waters. Float or swim around. The water draws out the pain and dissolves it. Feel the comfort. Stay in the water until you feel completely relaxed and comfortable. Swim back to the edge of the pond and walk out of the water, back across the clearing, back through the forest. You are feeling much better.

- Imagine floating down through layers of color. With each color you are enveloped in increasing relaxation and comfort. The first layer is golden-yellow. As you float down into the golden-yellow your unconscious is creating insight. The second layer is emerald-green. This layer relieves anxiety and instills a peaceful, calm feeling. Slowly drift down to a third layer that is indigo-blue. The indigo draws the pain out of your body and traps it, so that when you leave this layer, you leave all the pain behind. Float down into the next layer, which is a soft pink or lavender glow, immersing you in a feeling of love and comfort. The final layer is clear – a synthesis of all colors and a reminder of the balance necessary to a life of fulfillment.

- Relax as much as you can and focus on your breathing. Breathe slowly, so that each in-breath takes 3 to 4 seconds and each out-breath takes 3 to 4 seconds. Imagine that with each inhale, you are pulling soothing energy in through your feet and up through your body. As the energy moves upward through your body, it gathers up painful sensations along the way. As you exhale, imagine that the energy flows out of your body with your outward breath, letting the pain evaporate into the air. Repeat, as you notice subtle changes occurring in sensations of discomfort. With each inhale, silently say, "I breathe in comfort." With each exhale, silently say, "I breathe out discomfort."

Self-Hypnosis: Hypnotic Analgesia

Clinical hypnotherapists often teach hypnotic analgesia to patients in medical settings. It is a tried-and-true method for bringing numbness to pain. Here are the steps:

1. Apply any induction and deepening method of your choice.

2. Let one arm hang down off the side of your chair or bed. Make the arm loose and limp so that it dangles.

3. Imagine that your arm is immersed in a bucket of ice water. The water is freezing cold. Imagine chunks of ice floating in the water. Hear the ice chunks as they slosh around in the water and bump up against each other. Think about how cold your hand is getting in the

ice water. Colder and colder. The blood is withdrawing. Your hand is getting numb.

4. Remember a time when your hands felt cold and numb. You might remember playing or working outdoors in the winter, for example. Go into your memory of ice cold hands now, fully associated, so that you can bring back that cold, numb feeling in your hand.

5. Visualize that your hand is still in the cold bucket of ice water, getting colder and colder, getting so numb, there is no feeling in that hand whatsoever. Your skin takes on a leathery feeling. If you were to pinch the back of your hand with all your strength, that hand would feel nothing. No pain whatsoever.

6. Physically lift your hand and place it on the painful area. Imagine that your hand stays cold and numb. Imagine the cold numbness flowing into the painful area. Feel the pain receding as the icy numbness takes over.

7. Give yourself the suggestion that this numb feeling can continue for quite some time, even after you come out of self-hypnosis. Give yourself the suggestion that any time you touch this area with your "numbing" hand, in the future, the discomfort will shrink and recede, to be replaced with a comfortable, numb sensation.

8. Mental rehearsal: Visualize a future environment where you particularly want to feel comfortable. You hang your hand down into that imaginary ice bucket, letting it get very numb. Then you place your hand on the area of discomfort. The cold, numb sensation in your hand transfers into the area, bringing comfort.

9. Return your thoughts to the here and now. Say the affirmation, "I move and rest in ease and comfort" or devise an affirmation that you find suitable. Reorient.

Self-Hypnosis: Change the Submodalities of Pain

You'll recall from Chapter 3 that "submodalities" are elements of internal representations that we can manipulate to change meanings and perceptions. You can alter pain sensations by visualizing a representation of the pain, and then modifying the submodalities (i.e., the visual and kinesthetic elements). In effect, you are asking your brain to perceive pain in another way. There is no single formula for this process. In this self-hypnosis session, you'll experiment with several ways to alter your imagery to discover which modifications bring you the most relief or comfort.

1. Go into trance, using an induction and deepening method of your selection.

2. Visualize an image that represents your pain. It might be an object, or a three-dimensional geometric shape, or maybe just a blob. See the image outside your body, in your visual field. See the image as having dimensions, size, shape, substance, texture, and color. Often, this single step can bring comfort.

3. Experiment with changing the submodalities of the image, following the instructions below, to discover which changes bring more comfort. Go slowly through this process. Take time to notice the physical effects (what you feel in the painful area) of each change before moving on to the next one.

   • Begin with color. What color is your image? Change the color to another color – any other color you like. Pause for about 10 seconds while you continue visualizing the image in the new color. Breathe in comfort and breathe out discomfort. Sense any physical change. Change the image to yet another color. Pause about 10 seconds again while visualizing the image in the new color. Breathe in comfort and breathe out discomfort. Sense any change that occurs in your body.

   What is the effect of this second color? Change to other colors, one by one, to determine which color brings the most comfort. Breathe in comfort and breathe out discomfort. Welcome even small changes in sensations. Whatever color feels best, change the image to that color and keep it that color.

   • Visualize the size of the image. Make it smaller. Smaller is usually more comforting. Monitor your physical response. Experiment with varying sizes until you hit on one that seems to bring the most comfort. If you have no change in your physical response, just put the image back to the size it was originally. Breathe in comfort and breathe out discomfort.

- Distance is often a significant factor. Visualize the image as farther away – maybe across the room. Pause and monitor your physical response. Experiment with varying distances until you discover one that brings the most comfort. Keep the image at that distance. If you feel no change, bring the image back to where it was originally in your visual field. Breathe in comfort and breathe out discomfort.

- Location is another important aspect. Move your image to various locations in your visual field – up, down, left, and right. Let your eyes follow the image as it moves to each new location. After each move, pause to monitor your physical response. If you determine that one location brings more comfort, leave the image there. If you detect no change, bring the image back to where it was originally. Breathe in comfort and breathe out discomfort.

- Change the texture and apparent "substance" of the image. For example, if you originally imagined the pain as made of metal, change the substance to wood, paper, rubber, sponge, or gelatin. You might change a sheet of sandpaper to a soft baby blanket, for instance. As you change the substance, alter the surface texture accordingly. For each change, pause to notice associated physical changes. Breathe in comfort and breathe out discomfort.

- Think of any other changes in the image that might bring additional comfort. For example, if the image has sharp edges, make the edges rounded. You might rotate the image in space and view it from different angles. Each time you change the image, monitor your physical response. Maintain the changes that bring you the most comfort, no matter how subtle those changes might seem. Breathe in comfort and breathe out discomfort.

4. When you have changed the image sufficiently, suggest to yourself that your unconscious mind can memorize this final image and maintain it, even after you emerge from trance. Anticipate that you'll continue your day with improved ease and comfort.

5. Reorient and open your eyes.

Self-Hypnosis: Comfort Transfer

The Comfort Transfer method (also adapted from Bruce Eimer, mentioned earlier in this chapter) encourages you to concentrate on areas of the body that feel comfortable, with less attention to pain. Since this method includes imagery involving warmth, it might not be appropriate for pain that feels hot, burning, or feverish. Here are the steps:

1. Sit or recline comfortably. Induce trance and deepen with any method of your choosing.

2. Focus on any part of your body that feels comfortable. Notice the comfortable sensations. Breathe deeply and relax more with each exhale. With your breath, direct those sensations of comfort to areas that need more comfort. Imagine each in-breath as an energy that moves comfort around in your body. Allow the comfort to flow where you want it.

3. Affirmation: I breathe comfort from one part of my body to another.

4. Place your palm on your thigh. Become aware of the pulse in the fingertips of that hand. Feel that hand getting warm with the pulsing, drawing warmth from your thigh. When your hand feels sufficiently warm, place it on the affected part of your body. Spread the warmth into the area, bringing comfort. Imagine the warmth increasing, seeping into skin, muscles, and tissues.

5. Affirmation: I keep my hand on the pulse of growing comfort.

6. Give yourself the suggestion that your comfort will continue throughout the next few hours. Mentally rehearse an upcoming activity in which you participate with comfort and ease.

7. Reorient and open your eyes.

The Six D's of Pain Management

Bruce Eimer wrote that effective pain management relies on the six D's. I've summarized them below, explaining how they relate to self-hypnosis.

- **Deep relaxation:** Relaxation relieves the physical tension that often exacerbates pain. You can achieve deep relaxation through progressive relaxation, as you learned in Chapter 5. Affirmations of comfort and ease can also prove relaxing.

- **Decatastrophizing:** Catastrophizing means getting caught up in the anxiety of gloom-and-doom thinking. Decatastrophizing means that you develop the skills to pull yourself out of that kind of thinking. In this way, you keep your thoughts and emotions in check. Decatastrophizing uses logic and self-soothing thoughts to calm emotions.

- **Direction:** Direction is the process of guiding and directing your own thoughts and actions. Through self-hypnosis, you can use mental rehearsal and guided imagery to direct your thoughts in positive ways to instill hope and optimism. You can replace negative worry-thoughts with positive, uplifting affirmations.

- **Distraction:** Distraction directs your thinking away from pain toward other sensations such as comfort and relaxation. Distraction also means that you take your attention off of pain and direct it to other interests and activities. We've seen this occur in professional sports, where a player sustains a minor injury but is so involved in the game that he remains unaware of pain until after the game is over.

- **Distortion:** Distortion is a coping strategy that involves re-interpreting pain sensations, so that they mean something else. A mother giving birth interprets her pain as signalling the arrival of her child. For an athlete, sore muscles after a work-out might mean increased srength. Chronic pain often carries a psychosomatic message that, once acknowledged, allows the reduction of unnecessary pain. Used hypnotically, distortion actually changes how the brain interprets sensory input (pain). It makes pain easier to tolerate.

- **Dissociation:** Dissociation is a coping mechanism for disengaging from pain. In hypnosis, it means assigning the perception of pain to one's unconscious mind, so that the pain is unavailable to conscious awareness. While this may seem impossible, it is a fact that under hypnosis, some people have undergone abdominal surgery without any chemical anaesthesia, remaining awake and comfortable throughout the process. Hypnotic dissociation takes practice, but can be achieved so that pain management becomes easier and more automatic.

Explore the pain management strategies in this chapter to train your brain to ignore pain and seek comfort and pleasure. Tell your unconscious mind to devise safe tactics to discount familiar, unnecessary pain that conveys no new or significant information. Thank your unconscious for giving you increased freedom day by day.

Imagine going about your daily activities with reduced pain and increased ease and comfort. Imagine having a smile on your face as you tell a friend or loved one that your pain level has reduced since you learned self-hypnosis. Mentally rehearse enjoying life more, with less pain.

CHAPTER 18

Preparing for Surgery or Medical Procedures

It's understandable to feel anxious about surgery and medical procedures. These are often painful, the results may be uncertain, and for many, they mean a loss of personal control. Added to these concerns are worries about the long-term and short-term implications of illness. If you anticipate surgery, managing your stress levels is particularly important if your immunity has been compromised by illness or the side-effects of medications, drugs, or chemotherapy.

Prior to surgery, self-hypnosis will help you prepare mentally, lower anxiety, facilitate your body's optimum responses during surgery, and promote healing and recovery. Studies show that hypnosis, before and/or during surgery, speeds the healing of bone fractures as well as post-surgical wounds.[72] A study by the National Cancer Institute found that women undergoing surgery for breast cancer, who received a brief hypnosis session before surgery, required less anesthesia and pain medication during surgery.[73] They reported less pain, nausea, fatigue, and discomfort after surgery than women in a control group. The overall cost of surgery was also significantly less for women who had hypnosis.

Radiologist Elvira Lang led a study on 241 patients undergoing minimally invasive radiological procedures.[74] The patients were sedated, with no or minimal anesthesia. One third of the patients received hypnosis with guided imagery during surgery. One third received "attention" from a medical staff member trained in hypnosis, during surgery. The final one-third, the control group, underwent standard surgical procedures. The hypnosis group reported the least pain and had the least drug intake. Only one person in the hypnosis group had cardiovascular difficulty, compared to 12 in the control group. The procedure time averaged 61 minutes in the hypnosis group, compared to 78 minutes in the control group.

For most people, just one or two hypnosis sessions can significantly improve the outcome of surgery and the subsequent healing and recovery. Numerous studies published in medical journals show that, with hypnotherapy, less anesthesia is needed, operating times are shorter, and patients have fewer complications, less post-operative pain, and faster recovery. Hypnosis helps surgery patients feel relaxed and positive before, during, and after surgery.

In self-hypnosis prior to surgery or a medical procedure, you can give yourself many helpful suggestions as to your emotions and thoughts going into the procedure, physical responses during the procedure, and post-surgery recovery and healing. If you remain awake during the procedure, you can also use self-hypnosis to reduce anxiety and discomfort. Many women, for example, have gone through childbirth comfortably with hypnosis and guided imagery, instead of drugs.

Talk to Your Medical Team about the Value of Hypnosis

Some hypnotherapists are trained in "hypno-anesthesia," especially useful for surgical patients who do not tolerate chemical anesthesia. In fact, many hospitals now allow a clinical hypnotherapist into the operating room, at patient request. Depending on the procedure, many hospitals and clinics also allow patients to listen to hypnotic recordings during medical procedures. If you plan to listen to hypnotic recordings or hire a hypnotherapist, make arrangements with your medical team in advance. Many hospitals have a hypnotherapist on staff or your physician can recommend one.

If you plan to use self-hypnosis as preparation for surgery, talk to your surgeon in advance, explaining your plan. Ask what physical responses on your part would make for optimum conditions during the surgery. You can then incorporate those suggestions into your self-hypnosis sessions, to be fulfilled in the operating room. Your surgeon, for example, might prefer that you maintain a moderate blood pressure level, steady breathing and heart rate, minimal bleeding, and a normal body temperature. You can also give yourself suggestions that you will come out of surgery with minimum pain and swelling and that you will easily swallow liquids such as water or fruit juice and that your stomach will easily digest food. You can tell your body that it can begin healing immediately.

Inform your physician that he can speak to you during surgery to suggest desirable physical responses. You can suggest to yourself in self-hypnosis that, even though you will be asleep or heavily sedated in the operating room, your body will follow the instructions of the medical team, when those instructions are specifically addressed to you. Tell your medical team to say your name before giving you such instruction.

In *Love, Medicine and Miracles*, oncologist Bernie Siegel pointed out that even under general anesthesia, some patients do, nevertheless, respond to a surgeon's instructions to alter physical responses such as breathing, heart rate, blood pressure, body temperature, and bleeding.[75] The unconscious remains attentive even while the conscious mind sleeps.

Self-Hypnosis: Preparation for Surgery

The self-hypnosis session below incorporates a number of hypnotic methods covered elsewhere in this book, such as goal imaging, guided imagery, and mental rehearsal. The purpose is to help you prepare psychologically for surgery or a medical procedure. By feeling calm and self-assured before, during, and after the surgery or procedure, it's possible you'll achieve greater comfort and have a smoother recovery.

Remember, hypnosis does not replace your physician's instructions. It is an adjunct to your doctor's skill and recommendations. The self-hypnosis session below will also help you to trust your medical team, so that you can relax and let them do their job. It will also help you to remember that there is life after surgery. The way to overcome an anticipated difficulty is to remind yourself that you'll be glad when it's over. This generic script assumes a procedure involving anesthesia. Change the wording as needed to suit your individual circumstances. Here are the steps:

1. Induce and deepen trance using any method of your choice.

2. Speak to your body silently: calmly and gently explain to your body that it will soon undergo a medical procedure. Explain, in general,

what the procedure may involve, such as injections, drugs, sutures, and so on. Say that you have given permission for the procedure to take place, so that, in the long run, the body will be healthier, stronger, and have less discomfort. Say that the body will be in good hands. Tell your body that the procedure will be safe and helpful.

Tell your body that, on the day or the procedure, you'll feel calm and relaxed. Ask your body to readily accept anesthesia and/or any administered medications and tolerate them well. Remind your body that you intend for your heart rate, pulse, and blood pressure to stay steady, to help the medical team as they do their work. Your immune system is standing by, ready to marshal antibodies to dispose of any unwanted germs, viruses, or bacteria that aren't supposed to be there. Tell your body to follow the medical team's instruction, only if they speak to you directly. Tell your body that when the procedure is over, you'll be allowed to rest comfortably for a time.

3. Mental rehearsal: Visualize and anticipate that in the days leading up to the surgery you feel calm, with inner peace and contentment. You are in good spirits. You sleep well at night, falling asleep easily and waking up when you want to wake up, feeling awake and alert.

    On the morning of surgery you wake up feeling calm and serene. Your appetite has temporarily gone away. You appreciate all the people who are assisting you on this day. When you arrive at the hospital, you might find your contentment increases. You feel at ease asking questions of your medical team that might help to increase your equanimity and comfort. You realize the procedures will be over soon. By the end of the day, you'll be resting safe and sound.

    As you get prepped for surgery, ignore things you don't like and instead focus on whatever is most appealing and comfortable. You feel calm and serene. (Add any other suggestions or images that you might find helpful.) Gradually, you'll receive an injection and drift off into slumber.

    Later, you'll wake up in the recovery room, feeling safe and peaceful. You realize where you are. You feel comfortable and appreciative. You swallow liquids with comfort. In a little while you feel more alert.

Your appetite returns. You feel glad the surgery is over and recovery has begun.

4. Bless your medical team and their work. Bless their hands, their minds, and their skills. Feel gratitude for their expertise and training. They are helping you to get well. Trust that they will serve you well.

5. Goal imaging: Visualize your complete recovery. Imagine what you'll be doing with much more ease and comfort, perhaps more stamina or fortitude.

6. Bring your thoughts back to the here and now. Reorient and open your eyes.

Following surgery, you might find self-hypnosis additionally useful for pain management (see Chapter 17). In fact, you might want to record one or two scripts from Chapter 17 in advance of surgery to have ready for your recuperation and recovery.

Self-Hypnosis: A Healing Visualization

When your surgery or medical procedure is complete, you might want to practice the following healing visualization,[76] featuring a wisdom figure.

1. Induce and deepen trance with any method of your choosing.

2. Visualize a healing place; actual or imaginary. Visualize details such as color, lighting, textures, and so on. Imagine beautiful objects in this healing setting. You might also include pleasant sounds, temperatures, and fragrances.

3. Imagine a healing companion who joins you in your healing place. This companion might be a departed loved one, a guardian angel, a spirit guide, a historic healer, or a holy personage. Allow this companion to relate to you in comforting ways: Perhaps with words, poetry, or music. This companion might offer you a symbolic gift or surround you with love and light.

4. While your companion continues to comfort you, imagine a conversation with your body. First, thank your body for all it does it for you, day and night, without your having to remind it. It digests food, circulates blood, conducts elimination and respiration, and carries out hundreds of additional processes. Thank your body for its healing capabilities. Realize that your body has already begun the healing process. Realize that even though one part of your body may have sustained illness or damage, other parts continue to function quite well.

Second, remind your body about many other instances in the past when you were ill or injured, but your body healed and recovered. Remember how your body let you know it was getting well. Remember the pleasant discoveries about your body's ability to heal. Praise your body for its healing abilities and remind it to apply those abilities again, now.

5. Imagine a healing, comforting, protective glow surrounding your body, as the body activates it positive energies and internal wisdom. See this glow saturating your body tissues, down to the cellular level.

6. Affirmation: I have the ability to heal. I am confronting this challenge, to survive and to thrive.

7. Thank your healing companion. Ask your companion to continue to watch over you and monitor your healing, sending you comfort and healing intentions. Assume that your unconscious is memorizing the details of this healing place, to return to it again and again in the days and weeks to come. Say farewell to your healing companion for now.

8. Visualize a dissociated image of your self, in the future, well and active again. Know that your body holds the wisdom to recover on its own schedule.

9. Reorient and open your eyes.

This particular visualization can be adapted for children. Children can draw or paint pictures of themselves in a healing place, surrounded by family members and a healing wisdom figure. They can draw a picture of themselves surrounded by a healing glow. They can also make up songs and poems about leaving the doctor's office or hospital, resting, and getting better each day, and returning to normal activities.

In recovering from any illness or injury, keep in mind that thoughts influence the body. Do your best to maintain optimistic expectations. Your body will respond.

CHAPTER 19

Heal Emotional Hurts Connected with the Past

Time is ever-present and never-ceasing. We exist forever in the present but because of memory and imagination, our thoughts and emotions easily shuttle between past and future. Emotions and psychological well-being are often connected to our perceptions of past and future. Depending on what we are doing and how we are feeling, time seems to possess elasticity, speeding up or slowing down. We can focus on an activity to the extent that we lose track of time altogether. In hypnosis, we call it "time distortion."

Given that time is so much an element of our psychology, it's hardly any wonder that the early developers of NLP came up with strategies for working with personal time lines.[77,78] Time line interventions, mentioned in Chapter 3, are strategies that alter one's visual representations, on an imagined time line, to alleviate the negative effects of past events, enhance resourcefulness and problem-solving, and shape positive expectations. This chapter focuses on time-line trance-work.

A Brief History of NLP and Time Lines

Early on, the developers of NLP noticed that people looked in particular directions according to what they were thinking. They observed that most people look and gesture to their left when remembering the past and to the right when imagining future possibilities.[79]

NLP trainers Connirae Andreas and Steve Andreas combined the observation with the understanding that individuals experience remembered past events and anticipated future events in linear fashion. They noticed that people represent events in time in a visual-spatial manner called a time line. Past events are usually represented as lining up on the left or behind the body. Anticipated future events usually line up on the right or in front of the body. We do not locate our time lines inside our heads – we organize them *outside* our bodies! Additionally, most of us are not consciously aware of doing so.

Connirae Andreas observed that people have subtle kinesthetic responses to verb tenses.[80] If you represent these three sentences: "I danced," "I dance," and "I will dance," you'll have three distinct internal representations and three distinct sets of sensations. You'll "locate" these three representations at distinct points on your time line, representing past, present, and future. We do these things consistently and unconsciously.

NLP trainers started eliciting time lines, finding many individual variations. Although people consistently arrange their past, present, and future in a linear manner, the similarities stop there. Some are curved, some are straight, and some are looped. Some are still, while others seem to undulate or vibrate with energy. Some are narrow and some are wide with hills and valleys. Some have light and dark areas. Some time lines appear as symbols: a beam of light, a river, a road, or a stack of DVDs.

For some people, their "now" is right in front of the body, usually between eye-level and the waist. Sometimes "now" intersects the body. Where time lines begin and end is also fascinating. Some people see their time lines as beginning at birth or conception. Some see their time lines extending backward infinitely into past life incarnations. Some people see their future ending at death, while others see their time lines continuing after death into an afterlife or future incarnations.

The Andreas team observed that people could make lasting emotional and behavioral changes just by modifying the submodalities of their time line representations.[81] Altering the configuration, lighting, and colors of time lines could often bring about new perceptions, feelings, and even beliefs. They also found that time lines could serve as a backdrop for reframing past events and for anticipating future events in a resourceful way.

Moreover, people can imagine traveling their time lines in two ways. They can travel *on* their time lines, in an associated manner, like walking on a street. Conversely, they can visualize floating *above* their time lines, in a dissociated fashion, like floating in the air, moving parallel to the street. Discovering that individuals could navigate their times lines, NLP trainers developed therapeutic patterns to help people relate to the past, present, and future more resourcefully. Today, NLP practitioners apply time line strategies to a wide range of client problems.

Charting Your Time Line

Charting your time line is an intuitive process. Follow the instructions below. For each instruction, sit quietly and close your eyes, allowing images and feelings to emerge. If you think you are "making it up" that's okay – you are. The general position in NLP is that all of reality is made up!

Think about brushing your teeth this morning. Point to where you "place" that image. You'll probably be pointing somewhere outside of your body.

- **Chart your past time line:** For each of the following, point sequentially to various locations outside your body. Point to where you place thoughts about:
  - Brushing your teeth yesterday morning.
  - Brushing your teeth on the morning of the day before yesterday.
  - Something you did last week.
  - Something you did a month ago.
  - Something you did three months ago.
  - Something you did last year.
  - Something you did five years ago.

  Notice how all these past experiences line up. Connect the dots and trace your time line as it stretches into the past. Visualize your past time line.

- **Chart your future time line:** Think about brushing your teeth tomorrow morning. Point to where you store that thought. Think about the following sequentially and point to various locations outside your body. Point to where you store thoughts about:
  - Brushing your teeth two mornings from today.
  - Brushing your teeth three mornings from today.

- – Something you plan to do a month from now.
- – Something you plan to do three months from now.
- – Something you'll probably do one year from now.
- – Something you'll probably do five years from now.

Again, notice how all these future possibilities line up. Connect the dots to trace your time line into the future. Visualize your future time line.

- **Locate "now"**: Where is your "now?" Does it go through your body, or is it in front of you? How big is it? My experience is that most people like "now" to be about shoulder-width. Experiment with different sizes to find one you like.

- Visualize floating upward, slightly above your time line, looking down at it. Look it over, in both directions. Note the dimensions and configurations. Notice events lining up on your future time line. Look at one or more events on your past time line. Float over a planned future event and locate it. How do you imagine it? Float back over "now." Float over a recent past event. How do you represent it? Float back over "now" and down into it.

Now you are familiar with the layout of your time line and you know how to "travel" above it in a dissociated manner. Time line visualizations are so engrossing that most people easily go into trance with time line work. You are ready to move on to time line applications.

Precautions about Working with Hurtful Memories

The applications in this chapter are not intended to replace psychotherapy or psychiatric care. If you are troubled by the enduring effects of trauma, seek professional help rather than rely on the exercises in any self-help book. If particular memories of past hurtful events overwhelm you emotionally, do *not* choose those particular memories for the applications that follow. These applications are appropriate only for memories that the reader can tolerate emotionally.

The NLP approach to healing hurtful past events differs from that of therapies relying on regression and catharsis in which the individual must re-associate into the event in order to reach resolution, often re-experiencing the emotions. While cathartic therapies certainly have their successes, the NLP approach is to review hurtful events in a dissociated manner, with as much comfort as possible.

Healing a memory of a hurtful event does not erase the fact that it happened. Healing a memory in no way invalidates your feelings and responses at the time. In no way does it justify what happened. Even though you heal a memory, you would still retain the discoveries, insights, and strengths you might have acquired. The purpose of healing a memory is to neutralize the lingering negative effects.

Self-Hypnosis: Healing a Memory – Variation 1

This first variation on Healing a Memory takes you (via imagination) back over your time line to a point *before* a hurtful event, to send and receive healing intentions. Then you'll pass over the event and see yourself at the end of it. You will *not* access the hurtful event at all. You'll return to "now" and receive those healing intentions as they travel forward through time.

If your chosen memory includes a series of similar events (such as repeated bullying in the school playground), you'll float above your time line back to before the earliest incident and send and receive healing intentions. Then you'll float up above your time line and pass over all the similar events, until you reach the point where the last one is over and done. Once more, you'll send healing intentions. You'll return to "now" and receive those healing intentions coming forward in time.

Choose a memory of a hurtful event that exerts a negative influence today, at least in specific situations. If it was a series of similar hurtful events that exerted a cumulative effect, choose the first and last instance you remember. This application may help to heal the effects of that memory and to neutralize its negative influence. It's possible that you'll no longer feel discomfort when you recall the memory or when something reminds you of the event(s). If the event(s) has exerted a continuing detrimental effect on your emotions in specific situations then, from now on, in those situations, you will most likely have a more resourceful response.

This self-hypnosis session is based on a time line strategy called "The Minute Before." To begin, answer these two questions so that you can later assess your results.

- What negative effects of the event(s) do you experience today?
- Assuming you'll release the emotional effects of that event, what outcome would you anticipate? In other words, how would you know the change has taken place?

Here are the steps:

1. Induce and deepen trance in any manner of your choosing.

2. Situate yourself at "now" on your time line. Visualize floating up just above your time line, looking down at it. From that vantage point, locate the hurtful event(s) on your past time line. The event(s) might look like a small video clip, a dark shadow, or a storm cloud. However you represent the event(s) intuitively will be fine.

3. Travel backward, above your time line, until you hover above the beginning of the event(s). Look backward, just before the event took place. See an image of your younger self, on your time line, just before she had any inkling that something bad was going to happen.

4. As you visualize her, you know what is about to happen, but she doesn't. You also know that she will survive and when the event(s) will end. Send compassionate healing intentions for her benefit.

5. Float down into the time line and associate into the moment before the event begins. Bring the knowledge that you'll survive and that the ordeal will come to an end. You don't realize it yet, but having this small bit of knowledge ahead of time will make a difference, influencing how you process the event as it occurs and afterward. Receive the healing intentions.

Look forward in time to the end of the event(s). Send your healing intentions forward across your time line through the event(s), all the way to the end, and beyond the end point, forward to your "now."

6. Float back up above your time line, moving forward, quickly moving past the event(s), to the point at which the event(s) is over. Look down at the younger you who survived it. Send her additional healing intentions. Travel forward, above your time line, returning to "now." See your healing intention, like a beam of energy, also traveling forward toward you, on your time line.

7. When you arrive above "now," float down into "now," feeling the full force of the healing intention as it catches up with you, bringing positive, healing energy into your present. Look backward in time and see your past infused with healing energy. Send your healing intentions forward into your future time line, so that the healing effects continue indefinitely.

8. Mental rehearsal: Move forward on your time line, toward the outcome that you anticipate, now that you have healed the past. Be in that situation now, feeling free, more resourceful. Notice and enjoy the differences in your thoughts and feelings and possibly new actions. Float above your time line and return to "now," floating down into the present.

9. Return your thoughts to the here and now. Reorient and open your eyes.

From the NLP standpoint, time lines are visual metaphors. Realize that past events no longer exist, except in how we remember them. With time line trance-work we can change how we represent past events, so that our brains "recode" those memories.

Self-Hypnosis: Healing a Memory – Variation 2

Sometimes a memory is painful because we didn't get the care or support afterwards that would have made a difference in how we then remember the event. For example, if you fell and broke your leg on the street, and people just passed by, it would be a different experience from one in which someone stopped to help and stayed beside you until an ambulance arrived. Your emotional response to those two memories would be different, wouldn't they?

This variation on Healing a Memory asks you to consider how your emotional response to a hurtful memory could be different *today*, if someone had helped you *then*. Again, you'll identify a hurtful event that continues to exert a negative influence over your present, at least in specific situations. If it was a series of similar hurtful events that exerted a cumulative effect, choose the *last* instance you can remember, when the events finally came to an end.

In this application, you'll float over your past time line and visualize your younger self when a hurtful event(s) has come to an end. Sometimes the end point is difficult to determine because even though the event itself is over, the physical and/or emotional pain might continue for some time. Use your judgment on this. I usually say to my clients: "An event is 'over' when you are out of danger, others are out of danger, or in the case of loss, all that's left to do is grieve."

This time line application may help heal the effects of a painful memory, so it no longer exerts a negative effect. That means you'll no longer feel discomfort upon recalling the memory or when something reminds you of the event(s). If the event(s) has exerted a continuing detrimental effect on your emotions in specific situations, then from now on, in those situations, you'll most likely feel more resourceful.

This self-hypnosis strategy is based on a combination of NLP methods for healing the past. Before you begin, answer these two questions, which will help you assess your results.

- What negative effects of the event(s) do you experience today?

- If you could release the emotional effects of that event, what outcome would you anticipate? In other words, how would you know the change has taken place?

Here are the steps:

1. Induce and deepen trance with any method of your choosing.

2. Situate yourself at "now" on your time line. Float up above "now."

3. Float backward above your time line until you locate the hurtful event(s). The event(s) might look like a small video clip, a dark shadow, or a storm cloud. However you represent it intuitively will be fine. Locate the point on your time line (in the past) where the event(s) was over and done.

4. Look down. Visualize an image of your younger self, on your time line, after the event(s) is over and done.

5. Float down beside him, feeling kindness and compassion. Imagine that you and he look at each other. Reach out and hold his hand. He senses your kindness and compassion and it warms his heart, giving him resilience, strength, and hope, which he is not aware of at this time. Turn toward the past and hold your hand up to the event, like a policeman stopping traffic. Say to the event, "Stop! The influence stops here and now. I neutralize this event!" Turn away from the event, toward your younger self.

    Speak to him. Say, "You survived. You did the best you could. It was not your fault. That event is over now. It will not happen again. You can heal from this. I am here with you now. I give you my intentions for your healing." Say anything else to comfort him.

6. As you stand beside him, imagine now that your healing intention turns into a beam of glowing energy, flowing out from your heart to his. The energy expands until it turns into a globe of light, enveloping the two of you. The light transforms into energies of healing and resilience.

7. Let your bodies merge. Holding on to that healing energy, travel forward quickly across your time line, back to "now." As you travel, healing energy infuses every memory and every experience. Moving

at the speed of thought, return to "now." Look back. See the past infused with healing energy.

8.   Mental rehearsal: Move forward on your time line, toward your outcome, now that you have healed the past. Be in that situation now, feeling free and more resourceful. Notice and enjoy the differences in thoughts and feelings, and possibly new actions. Float above your time line and return to "now," drifting down to the present.

9.   Return your thoughts to the here and now. Reorient and open your eyes.

Sometimes it's difficult to release the effects of negative experiences because of convictions such as, "It shouldn't have happened in the first place" or "I'm to blame because I shouldn't have been there/done that in the first place." What's done is done. Maybe it *shouldn't* have happened, but it did. Maybe you could have done something different, or maybe not. No one goes through life unscathed and without regrets. You can't change the past by holding on to it.

Self-Hypnosis: Bring a Resource Forward in Time

Fictional accounts tell charming, intriguing, and fascinating stories of people who travel in time. *A Christmas Carol*, to me, remains the classic time travel story. Scrooge refuses to celebrate Christmas. Then, in a dream, he meets three spirits: the ghosts of Christmas Past, Christmas Present, and Christmases Yet to Come. Each spirit shows him events of the past, present, and a possible future, respectively. With each event, Scrooge learns something that changes his outlook and his charity toward others. Apparently, Dickens knew a thing or two about time lines and wisdom figures!

In this self-hypnosis session, inspired by NLP trainer Robert Dilts, you'll meet wisdom figures on your time line.[82] The goal is to identify a personal resource that you want more of in the future. It should be a trait such as confidence, motivation, discipline, poise, patience, concentration, and so on. Decide now what resource you want to enhance, and the circumstances in which you want it. Your outcome, for example, might be "to have more confidence in public speaking" or "to listen more patiently to my customers."

In self-hypnosis, you'll retrieve this resource from a past experience, bring it forward into the present, and project it into the future. At each point in your time line – past, present, and future – you'll be guided by pairs of wisdom figures.

Use your imagination to choose your six wisdom figures. In every case, the wisdom figure you visualize should feel and express benevolent kindness toward you. These wisdom figures could be ancestors, spiritual entities, fictional characters, celebrities, or historic figures. Each will give you guidance and encouragement for accomplishing your outcome. Wisdom figures help us to access intuitive ideas and insights that we might not have thought of otherwise. For convenience, I'll refer to the wisdom figures with the numbers 1 to 6. Here are the steps:

1. Induce and deepen trance in any manner you choose.

2. Situate yourself on your time line at "now." Float up above your time line. Looking backward, toward the past, locate a memory in which you demonstrated the desired resource to your satisfaction. It could be a pleasant memory or a memory in which you demonstrated your resource in a problematic situation.

3. Float over your time line until you arrive at the location of the memory you identified in Step 2. Float down into the memory. Be there, accessing the resourceful state. Replicate the sights, sounds, thoughts, and emotions. When you are sure you have re-activated the resourceful state, hold on to it, letting it continue, as the context fades away.

4. Imagine now, two wisdom figures standing on either side of you on your time line, in this past moment. Look at Wisdom Figure 1, who speaks to you. Listen to her words – something that helps you to hold on to this resource. Let the words sink in. Repeat this process for Wisdom Figure 2. Send the energy of your resource forward in time, into "now," like a beam of light.

5. Bring your resource forward, along your time, traveling back to "now." Be aware of having this resource in the present. Again, imagine two wisdom figures standing on either side of you on your time line. Look at Wisdom Figure 3, who speaks to you. Listen to his words – something that helps you to intensify this resource, accessing it more fully. Let the words sink in. Repeat this process for Wisdom Figure 4. Send the energy of your resource forward in time, into your future, like a beam of light.

6. Move forward into the future, bringing the resourceful state. Stop at a point in which you imagine accessing that resource consistently and reliably, in a variety of contexts where it is most useful. Again, imagine two wisdom figures standing on either side of you. Look at Wisdom Figure 5, who speaks to you. Listen to what she says – something that helps you to intensify this resource, making it possible to access this resource whenever you intend to. Let the words sink in. Repeat this process for Wisdom Figure 6. Send the energy of your resource forward in time, into your future, so that it continues on, like a beam of light.

7. Imagine instances in this future in which you are accessing your resource. Think of where you'll be and what you'll be doing, thinking, saying, and feeling. Enjoy the pleasure, satisfaction, and rewards of consistently demonstrating this resource. Look backward to "now" and let your unconscious reverse engineer all that you did, from then until now.

8. You are on your future time line, in the role of your future self. Look back to "now" and see your present-day self looking forward at you. You know the satisfaction of having the resource. Say something meaningful to your present-day self that will give her help and encouragement in accomplishing the outcome. See how she accepts your message.

9. Return to "now" and take the place of your present-day self. Look ahead to the future and see your future self. Listen again to her words of encouragement. Receive them and let them uplift you. Still in the resourceful state, project it forward again, across your time line, doubling its potency into your future.

10. Replay all the messages from the wisdom figures. Let these messages support your intention. Anticipate how good it will be to easily access your resourceful state from now on. Bring your thoughts back to the here and now. Reorient and open your eyes.

Why does it help to send resources forward in time or to mentally rehearse having them? Because the present is a platform for imagining future possibilities. The future begins in the now.

Another Way of Thinking about Trauma

While we cannot change the "facts" of past events, we can always change how we now think about those events. We can declare that the pain of the past is over and release it. Years ago, I read about an international survey of trauma survivors. The survey asked the subjects how trauma had changed their lives. One third of the respondents said the quality of their lives had been diminished by trauma. One third said their lives had been disrupted, but eventually their lives returned to the same quality as before. The final third said that having survived trauma gave their lives a deeper, richer meaning. How is that possible? I believe they found within the experience of trauma new understandings about human nature, perhaps gratitude and spiritual insights.

Some years ago, I attended a training program in Rapid Trauma Resolution® by hypnotherapist Jon Connelly, an innovative therapist and trainer living and practicing in Florida. He told an entrancing teaching tale that offers another way to think about the hurtful experiences in our lives. I found the metaphor so meaningful, I couldn't forget it. I'd like to share it with you, as I remember it, and in my own words.

> Imagine taking a Sunday drive across the desert to visit a friend who lives within a day's drive. You travel alone. Midway through the drive, your car breaks down. You can't fix your car or restart it. You wait hours for help to come, but none arrives. You try to call with your cell phone, but there's no signal. You're stranded, surrounded by desert, with no food or water. It grows dark. You spend the night in your car.
>
> The next morning, you wake up hungry and thirsty, realizing you will die if you wait for help that may never arrive. You set out by foot

in the direction of the nearest town. You walk for hours in the searing heat. You grow weak, hungry, and thirsty. Soon you can no longer walk, but you crawl on your hands and knees, across the burning sands. Your skin is red and blistered. You wonder if you'll survive. At times you don't think you can go on. Night comes. You sleep on the cold sand, shivering. The next morning, you set out again, struggling with every step, sometimes crawling, nearly delirious with thirst and hunger.

Finally, in the distance, you see a town. You trudge onward, near total collapse. As you come to the outskirts of the town, you see a street with shops and people. You are too tired to call out, so you stagger on. People stare, not knowing what to do.

Then, you see one thing that you want more than anything else. You see a fountain of clear, cool water. Ignoring all else, you use your last bit of energy to reach that fountain. You want that water so much! The fountain is just meters away. Now it's just a few steps away. Now all that delicious, cool water is within your reach!

What do you do next? Do you plunge your hands and face into the cool, refreshing water and gulp it down, overwhelmed with joy and gratitude that your ordeal is over ... or do you curse the desert?

CHAPTER 20

Access Your Intuitive Wisdom

Intuition consists of understandings and ideas that we acquire spontaneously without a logical or analytical process. It seems to emerge from a source of which we are not consciously aware. You could say it comes from the unconscious mind.

We experience intuition in hunches, dreams, creativity, and in a sudden insight. We sometimes experience intuition when we are so in sync with another that we know what he or she is thinking. We can experience intuition as a thought or as a feeling, or both.

Intuition is at play when we find meaning in coincidences – something the renowned psychiatrist Carl Jung (1875–1961) called "synchronicity." In fact, Jung suggested that intuition might draw information from a wider field of consciousness all around us – the Collective Unconscious.

While many psychics are probably highly intuitive, being intuitive is not about being psychic. Being intuitive doesn't mean you'll predict the next World Cup championship team. Accessing your intuition is about discovering information for making decisions, figuring out the "next step" in a project, healing and health, insight into relationship issues, interpreting dreams, and for general problem-solving. With intuition, you can sometimes know just what to say or do to reach out to another in a helpful way. Intuition will assist you to get in sync with the wisdom around you and within you.

Tips for Success with Intuition

In this chapter, you'll learn self-hypnosis strategies for accessing your intuition, to obtain guidance about a problem or concern. These strategies are particularly useful for those difficult issues where it seems there is no one right answer. Here are some tips for a rewarding experience.

- Keep your mind open, receptive, non-judgmental, and curious. Stay in the moment as much as possible. Trust your feelings and inner representations.

- Flow with the experience rather than directing it, analyzing it, or critiquing yourself.

- Keep a journal of insights and guidance. In this way, you'll begin to notice patterns and consistencies. You'll gradually feel more confident in your ability, as well as more trusting of your intuition. Journaling will help you to validate the information through hindsight and the passage of time.

- Understand that intuitive guidance might come to you all at once, or piecemeal, over several days.

- Understand, additionally, that instead of getting the answer you seek during your self-hypnosis session, you might be led to the answer over the course of the next few days. You might, for example, feel inclined to pick up a book, watch a television program, or speak to a friend, at which point you discover the answer you've been searching for. I think this happens because you've set the intention in your mind, and now your attention is unconsciously directed to whatever might prove helpful.

One caveat: I cannot guarantee the accuracy of the information you'll receive because your responses will be dependent on your mood and physical state at that moment. My advice is to experiment with the methods here and adapt those with which you feel most comfortable.

When you receive intuitive guidance, you might experience it is as an internal image (possibly a metaphor or symbol), voice, music, or a feeling. Some describe it as a "knowing" or a "hunch." You don't always have to be in trance to obtain intuitive guidance. Sometimes, all it takes is to sit quietly and listen to the whispering, sincere voice within. Sometimes all it takes is to trust what your feelings tell you.

Self-Hypnosis: Intuitive Guidance Method 1 – Message in a Memory

Suppose you could ask your unconscious to sort through your memories and select one that holds a message suitable for solving a present-day problem. This is a method for getting "unstuck." The Message in a Memory seems to offer insightful guidance, based on intuition. Choose an issue or a question you've been wrestling with. Here are the steps:

1. Induce and deepen trance with any method of your choosing.

2. Ask your unconscious to choose a memory that offers an insight or an answer to your concern. Let this memory emerge spontaneously in your conscious awareness. Review the memory.

3. Bring your thoughts and attention back to the here and now. Appreciate that your unconscious presented this memory to you.

4. How does the memory relate to your present-day concern? What is the message?

5. Anticipate how you will use the message. Reorient and open your eyes.

Self-Hypnosis: Intuitive Guidance Method 2 – Consult a Wisdom Figure

In Chapter 4, I introduced the concept of wisdom figures in hypnotic imagery. Some people conceive of wisdom figures as figments of the imagination; a metaphoric conduit for communication with the unconscious. Still others say that in representing wisdom figures, especially spiritual entities (saints, angels, and holy people), we are actually tapping into the consciousness of those beings through morphic energy fields.

If you'd like to consult wisdom figures or spirit beings for guidance, you can follow a two-part process. First, mentally construct (visualize) an inner sanctuary in which to meet your wisdom figure. It can be a natural setting or an indoor setting, based on fantasy or reality. Make the surroundings beautiful and soothing. It can house your favorite things – animals, flowers, art, music, books, furnishings, and even magical equipment. If you like, sketch your sanctuary on paper to visualize it more clearly. Get ideas from photos of natural vistas or rooms in interior design magazines.

Consulting with wisdom figures in your sanctuary is the second step of the process. Choose wisdom figures or spirit guides best suited to provide the assistance you seek. You can speak with an individual or a panel. Your wisdom figures can be fictional characters, historical personages, ancestors, celebrities, departed loved ones, experts, or even animals. Spirit guides might be angels, prophets, or saints. You can even ask your unconscious to surprise you with the perfect entity to respond to your concerns.

In consulting with guides or wisdom figures, don't guess the answers or role play. Present your concerns with honest curiosity and an open, receptive mind. Receive the answers patiently. Some sessions will be more productive than others, depending on your physical and emotional state and degree of concentration.

The answers you receive could be expressed in words, song, poetry, scripture, familiar quotations, or gestures. The wisdom figure or spirit guide might show you pictures or direct you to a source of additional information, such as a book or movie. It's been my experience that these "visitors" never give me more information than I can digest in one setting. The information I seek often arrives progressively, across several encounters. In self-hypnosis, consulting with wisdom figures or spirit guides follows these steps:

1. Induce and deepen trance with any method of your choosing.

2. Visualize your inner sanctuary. Invite in a wisdom figure or spirit guide.

3. Converse with the visitor. Present your concerns. Listen patiently for guidance. Ask for clarification as needed. At the end of the conversation, thank your visitor and say farewell. Prepare to leave your sanctuary.

4. Return your thoughts to the here and now. Anticipate how you will use the information you received. Reorient.

Self-Hypnosis: Intuitive Guidance Method 3 – Interpret a Dream

Do you think dreams are a communication from the unconscious? Many people do, including Robert Moss. In *Conscious Dreaming*, Moss, a shaman and professor of philosophy, wrote that dreams are spiritual tools through which we can anticipate the future, receive intuitive guidance, and resolve unfinished business.[83] Moss recommended keeping a dream diary to understand the symbols, patterns, and themes of dreams. He advised his readers to ask: What does my dream want me to know? What does my dream want me to do? You can also use self-hypnosis to interpret a dream. Here are the steps:

1. Induce and deepen trance with any method of your choosing.

2. Visualize your inner sanctuary (see above). Bring forth a "mental screen" – something like a television screen. Watch your dream (or whatever parts you remember) on the screen. Pick out three to five of the most salient characteristics: objects, people, sounds, feelings, or events. When you've watched the dream, put the screen aside.

3. Invite into your sanctuary a wisdom figure who can best help you interpret the dream. Welcome the wisdom figure. Ask what each element of the dream means. Ask "What is the message of this dream?" and "How does this dream apply to my present-day life?"

4. Listen patiently for the reply. Ask for clarification where needed. Thank the wisdom figure and say farewell. Prepare to leave your inner sanctuary.

5. Return your attention to the here and now. Anticipate how you will apply the information you have received. Reorient and open your eyes.

By the way, you can ask your unconscious to program your dreams. Before you go to sleep, select any troublesome issue. Ask your unconscious mind to produce a dream with some bearing on the issue. When you wake in the morning, journal about your dream. Note the significant objects, events, and people in the dream. Then use the strategy above to interpret the dream.

Another way to interpret a dream is to imagine yourself in the role of each object, event, and person in the dream. I found this idea in Patricia O'Hanlon-Hudson's charming little book: *Making Friends with Your Unconscious Mind*.[84] In each role, give a message to yourself. For example, suppose you have a dream that you are walking on a path and you rest under a tree. You would then say, "I am the path. My message is ..." and "I am the tree. My message is ..."

Additionally, notice puns, double meanings, metaphors, and symbols, and interpret those as well. It's more productive to figure out what these phenomena mean to you personally, rather than to consult a book on dream symbolism. Your unconscious mind will create symbols based on your individual history. According to Moss, it's often helpful to share your dream with another, and ask, "If you had this dream, what would it mean to you?" Sometimes when we hear another's input, it helps us to understand our dreams from another perspective.

Moments of Inspiration

Sometimes in moments of quiet contemplation we have deep insights when, it seems, we achieve a heightened awareness of our own capacities and the world around us. Some people say intuition is the language of the soul, opening our minds to new dimensions of reality. Sometimes we feel the spiritual presence of another – a deceased loved one or a guardian spirit. Sometimes these experiences are moments of enlightenment and knowledge.

Many inventions and scientific discoveries are the result of an intuitive "flash of genius" that accompanies daydreaming, waking up after a dream, or quiet contemplation. The story of Nikola Tesla (1856–1943) provides an example. As an engineer, he had always wanted to harness the power of Niagara Falls to convert it into electricity that could power homes, stores, schools, hospitals, and factories. While employed by Thomas Edison, he had his "eureka" moment. One evening, at twilight, in 1883, while feeding pigeons in a park, he had a vision of a vast, oscillating universe made of energy frequencies. He proceeded to develop the Tesla Coil that vibrated at 60 cycles per second – the perfect speed to produce alternating current.

Don't dismiss or ignore your intuitive moments. Honor them for the possibilities they may hold. My friend and colleague, the Reverend Prentice Kinser III, discussed paranormal and intuitive experiences in his book *Limitless Living*.[85] He gave his readers three ways to test the "truth" of spiritual or intuitive guidance:

- First, compare your intuitive guidance to "prior revelation." This means that you can trust the guidance you receive if it is consistent with the historical traditions of your faith and your values concerning morality, ethics, and safety.

- Second, discuss your message, interpretation, or revelation with a trusted mentor or spiritual advisor. Ask your advisor to evaluate your guidance in the light of common sense and rational thought.

- Third, test your guidance against your own gut feelings. True knowledge brings a sense of joy and peace.

CHAPTER 21

Define Your Life Purpose

I wrote this book to help readers confront a common human dilemma: we say we want to do one thing, but we do another. We keep doing things we don't like doing. Now, I'm going to say something controversial that some readers will not want to hear. I believe many of our unwanted habits and self-sabotaging behaviors mask our unacknowledged conflicts about defining and pursuing a purposeful life. By worrying, obsessing, and focusing attention and energy on compulsions, habits, addictions, procrastination, anger, anxiety, and feeling victimized, we avoid life's biggest question: What is my purpose?

Our self-imposed limitations may be attempts to distract ourselves from the fear that without drama, life would be empty and meaningless. I believe one of humanity's deepest core values is to live meaningfully. One of England's most inspirational writers, James Allen (1864–1912), put it succinctly: "You will become as small as your controlling desire; as great as your dominant aspiration."[86] If we define a purpose for living, we find that daily activities take on a new richness.

So let me ask: What is your purpose? Your life will feel incomplete until you have an answer. For some, it's a scary question. Some people hesitate to define their purpose because they fear others will disapprove. It could mean change and sacrifice. Devoting one's life to an overriding passion could mean forsaking other, less important activities – maybe even those in which one has made a considerable investment of time and money. For some, it means giving up the illusion of being a victim. It would mean making tough decisions and standing by them. It would mean believing in a pursuit so breath-taking, it's impossible to imagine doing anything else, no matter what the price.

Is it worth it? Yes. Here's why: define your purpose, live it, and you will then eliminate about 90 percent of self-sabotage. You will know very clearly what matters most and what you can dispense with or ignore. You will know what absolutely stirs your passion and energizes you. You will get out of your own way and love your life. You will come to terms with yourself as a human being with glorious accomplishments and massive shortcomings, and you will keep going, regardless. When you identify your purpose, it will drive you and you will get really clear on what your life is all about.

Therapist, life coach, and author Bill O'Hanlon recently produced an audio CD entitled *Let Your Soul Be Your Pilot: Finding Your Direction in Life*.[87] In it, he said that we can determine our life purpose in three ways: through our wounds, our anger, and our bliss. These are life's way of grabbing us by the lapels and shouting, "This is what you are supposed to do!" Let's examine each one.

- Our wounds are losses, failures, and hurts. Yet, in our emotional and physical injuries, we often find strength. Suffering can reveal the truth of who we are. Some find that their lives are diminished by trauma. Others find their lives enriched with a deeper meaning and purpose.

- What gets you angry? Through anger, we acknowledge inequity and injustice. We then transform anger into energy in support of a worthy cause. Like propulsion fuel, anger can launch a quest for justice; a mission to redress a wrong.

- When we do what we love, we follow our bliss. O'Hanlon's advice is to decide what activities bring us inspiration and happiness. Bliss points the way to the soul's calling.

Having purpose doesn't mean life will always be rosy. It only means that life becomes more rewarding and meaningful. It does mean that you no longer feel hopeless when things go wrong. You realize that the meaning of negative events in your life is not who to blame, or how much you hurt, but what you can do to heal and how you respond to the calling in the event. Living your purpose means that you make decisions based on authenticity and integrity with your values, rather than on pleasing others.

It's often the case that the people we most admire are driven by an overriding purpose. At the lowest points in their lives, they find strength and a noble commitment to their values. History is full of such people. Who do you admire? List their names. You'll find your soul whispering, "They are showing you the way!"

When you know your purpose and live it, you see your life journey from a new perspective. You'll find you are no longer buffeted by every mishap. You no longer shy away from the challenge to do your best. Here are a few questions that might help you identify your purpose:

- What challenges have I overcome? What is the calling in these challenges?

- What personal wounds have I healed? What have I learned from suffering?

- What strengths do I now possess?

- What is my talent or gift?

- What are the things I really love to do?

- What do others most admire about me?

- What wrong or injustice do I detest?

- What can I contribute to make the world a better place?

Traveling the Mythic Hero's Journey

All cultures have their legends of the hero's journey. The world's major religions were founded on the life and teaching of iconic figures who demonstrated a purity of purpose and gave their followers a life-transforming message. Our favorite stories are those about people who pursue a passion or champion a cause. They struggle against obstacles. They acquire skill and demonstrate courage. Their triumph is to live a life of integrity. Our heroes may be fictional or real. They represent an ideal. Their struggles and triumphs touch our hearts and teach us how to live authentically. Their lives are the stories of the mythic hero's journey.

In *The Hero's Journey*, NLP trainers Stephen Gilligan and Robert Dilts suggested that thinking of life as a heroic journey transforms us.[88] We identify our calling. We see that self-sabotage is only resistance to realizing our potential. Misfortunes are a spiritual message to acquire strength, skill, compassion, and forgiveness, and to release what we no longer need. Through difficulties and obstacles we discover life's intrinsic meanings. We realize that we are spiritual consciousness in human form.

Gilligan and Dilts characterized the journey as having these turning points:

- **The calling:** Life seems to be going along in a routine way. We might have a vague feeling that there has to be something more, but we don't know what it is. Then something disrupts the status quo. It might be a challenge, a crisis, an epiphany, an injury, or a loss. We recognize a need that only we can fulfill. We might discover a passion or a gift we've never known. Our soul is calling us to a purpose or mission. Responding takes dedication and courage to grow and evolve.

- **Refusal:** We turn away from the calling, fearing the sacrifices. We aren't ready. We find distractions. We procrastinate. Others may dissuade us because they think our calling is wrong. The soul creates havoc.

- **Crossing the threshold:** We make the commitment. We forsake our comfort zone and begin the journey. We undertake the task and respond to the calling we can no longer ignore. This is the point of no return. Our capabilities are challenged. We feel disconcerted, afraid, confused, uncertain, anxious, and paralyzed. At times we think about turning back or quitting, yet we go on.

- **Finding guardians:** We discover teachers, sponsors, coaches, and messengers to support us. Through our guardians, we learn how to walk the path we've chosen. We develop gifts, talents, and skills.

- **Facing shadows and demons:** People and circumstances oppose us. We encounter doubts, fears, and temptations – our shadows. We might revert to old unwanted habits or sink into addictions, personal neglect, or depression – our inner demons. The challenge is to come to terms with the shadows, face the demons, and renew commitment to the calling.

- **Developing an inner self:** Through emotional growth and spiritual wisdom, we learn to live our beliefs, values, and integrity. We pursue spiritual practices.

- **The transformation:** We develop resources through struggle, setbacks, failures, dedication, and battle. We live on purpose. We accomplish the task.

- **The return home:** We share our gifts with others. We are now guardians to others on their journeys.

The hero's journey is a process of evolving one's potential and unfolding one's spirit.

What follows are three self-hypnosis exercises to help you to: (1) define your soul's dream, (2) consult your guardians about the meaning of a problem, and (3) align with your purpose. These self-hypnosis strategies are adapted from Gilligan and Dilts, and others, and they are chosen to reflect elements of the mythic hero's journey.

Self-Hypnosis: What is Your Soul Dream?

In 2003, I read an article by counselor/coach Rue Anne Hass, describing an intuitive method for answering the question: What is your Soul Dream?[89] I noticed how easily her strategy could be adapted to self-hypnosis. It is based on viewing your life from various perspectives. I thought it summed up an ideal way of intuitively defining one's purpose. Here are the steps for this remarkable process:

1. Induce and deepen trance with any method of your choice.

2. From your own viewpoint, review your day-to-day life. Be aware of your strengths and weaknesses, joys and sorrows, and usual responses to people and events, both positive and negative.

3. Visualize that you drift out of your body and off to the side. Take the position of an observer, watching your day-to-day life without judgment.

4. Drift to a higher overview. Take the position of a wise mentor or a guardian angel – perhaps a "higher self." Look at your life through the eyes of this being who knows your strengths and weaknesses, limitations and difficulties. This being completely loves you, honors you, respects you, and wants the best for you. Answer the question: "What is the Soul Dream of the person I am watching? What is the deepest yearning that could shape this person's life?"

5. Visualize now, in whatever way feels right, that you are the World itself. Imagine the consciousness of the World as a being in the community of the cosmos, with challenges, yet with a powerful, loving intention to integrate all its richness and dramatic diversity into a harmonious whole.

    Be the World and watch that human identity (you) going through day-to-day life. Imagine that you (as the World) have called that human being to yourself, to incarnate and live here to express the unique quality or story contained in her Soul Dream. How does that person, in all her richness of who she is, benefit the World in a way that only she can do? How does her presence honor and awaken something in the life of the World?

    What images, words, thoughts, feelings, and intuitions come to mind as you hold these questions inside?

6. Return to your body. What answers have come to mind? Consider the wisdom you have acquired from these different perspectives. How does your Soul Dream define your purpose?

7. Reorient and open your eyes.

We are all in this universe to make a contribution. We are given intuition to examine our lives and discover a purpose. We can look around and notice what is wanted and needed that fits with what our intuition tells us we are destined to do.

244

Self-Hypnosis: Confront a Challenge with Spiritual Companions

Spiritual companions travel beside us on our life journey. They are teachers, friends, family members, and colleagues who support us, teach us, set an example, and challenge us. Some people would also add guardian angels and departed loved ones to the list. Our spiritual companions call upon us to access our potentials and remain true to our callings. In this self-hypnosis strategy, you'll imagine you are surrounded by a community of such companions.

You'll ask them about a challenge or an issue that you face that seems to block you from discovering or achieving your life purpose. It might be a financial setback, a relationship problem, or a form of opposition. It might be doubt, fear, or a temptation. Whatever the challenge, this self-hypnosis session will help you to see, within it, a calling from your soul. Here are the steps:

1. Induce and deepen trance with any method of your choosing.

2. Think about a challenge or issue you are facing.

3. Call forth your companions. Visualize that they are surrounding you, providing love and comfort, in the midst of your struggle.

4. Ask your companions:

    - What is my soul's positive intention in bringing about this challenge?
    - What is this challenge calling me to become or do or have?
    - What resources and understandings shall I bring to this challenge?

    After each question, wait patiently and intuitively receive answers from your companions. Ask for clarification if needed. Do not argue or analyze the answers. Accept whatever answer you receive and thank your companions.

5. Ask your companions how the problem reflects on your life purpose or calling.

6. Anticipate how you will apply this information in the coming days as you continue to confront the issue or problem.

7. Return your attention to the here and now. Reorient.

Self-Hypnosis: Align with Your Intention or Purpose

For this self-hypnosis strategy, have an intention to accomplish a task or a goal, or your overall life purpose. This method will help you align more completely with your intention or purpose. Here are the steps:

1. Induce and deepen trance with any method of your choosing.

2. State your intention or purpose as an affirmation.

3. Let images swirl through your mind, showing you resources that you bring to your intention or purpose. Let the images represent talents, skills, knowledge, creativity, experience, and emotional support. Feel gratitude for these gifts.

4. Extend your mind into the world around you, as though you are sending out the frequency of your intention or purpose, and finding matching energies that resonate with the frequency of your purpose or intention.

5. Sense that you are creating a magnetic field that brings you these matching energies in the form of ideas, support, connections, and opportunities. Receive whatever is coming to you at this moment. It might be a feeling, an idea, a word, a melody, an image, or a symbol. Let your mind absorb this gift, knowing that it will be incorporated into your knowledge base.

6. Goal imagery: See yourself in the future. Visualize that you are acting on your intention and/or fulfilling your purpose. See it, feel it, and know it.

7. Reorient and open your eyes.

When you align with your soul's calling, pursuing your purpose, creativity flows through you as though you are a conduit. You can approach difficulties more congruently because you are clear about where and how to invest your time, talents, and energies.

The Premises of the Hero's Journey

Gilligan and Dilts put forth the premise that humans are spirit embodied in physical form. Through our nervous systems, we experience individuality and consciousness. Life is a journey of spirit unfolding. As a manifestation of spirit, each of us is here to answer a calling and define a purpose. Addictions and self-destructive habits are an indication that we are resisting the unfolding of spirit within ourselves.

Transforming resistance and the dark shadows within ourselves is our greatest challenge. Not doing so creates negative energy and debilitating emotions. The gift of human consciousness is to transmute suffering and sorrow into happiness and wholeness. Life continually challenges us, so that we cannot rest on our laurels. Each time we move through a challenge and grow, we are better prepared for the next one.

People will oppose us and test our commitment to our calling. They will disregard our unique gifts and talents. Some will not care about us one way or another. Our misfortunes are a spiritual calling to acquire strength, skill, compassion, and forgiveness and to release what we no longer need.

I am reminded of Viktor Frankl (1905–1997). In *Man's Search for Meaning* he wrote of his seven-year ordeal in the concentration camps of Nazi Germany.[90] Witnessing and observing suffering and atrocities, he came to terms with the ultimate meaning of life. Speaking of himself and his fellow prisoners, he wrote: "We had to learn ... that it did not really matter what we expected from life, but rather what life expected from us. We needed to stop asking about the meaning of life and instead to think of ourselves as though we were being questioned by life."

Afterword

The difficulties, challenges, and responsibilities of daily life are enough to manage, without the frustrations of unwanted habits and performance anxiety. It is my hope that this book has given you the tools and strategies for ending the behaviors you don't want, and for replacing them with behaviors and thought patterns that are far more productive, rewarding, and satisfying.

This book has provided the following:

- Five ways to visualize solutions to everyday problems.
- Six ways to induce your own trance.
- Forty self-hypnosis strategies for specific applications.
- Dozens of tips to manage the common problems of living.

If you have a problem not covered in this book, go back and review Chapter 4. Imagining the accomplishment of a goal or a solution and mentally rehearsing the actions you can take may prove helpful. You may also find that you can modify the self-hypnosis processes in this book for problems that are similar to yours.

As you become adept with self-hypnosis, you'll find that it's not necessary to do a formal trance induction and reorientation, as I've described in Chapter 5 and on the accompanying CD. You'll find you can slip in and out of trance easily and quickly. You'll also find that you become more intuitive and creative at problem-solving, just by gaining familiarity with the structure of NLP strategies.

Roger Walsh, professor of psychiatry and behavioral sciences at the School of Medicine of the University of California, Irvine identified seven "wisdom traditions" that take the mind beyond ordinary waking awareness.[91] When people systematically train their minds through wisdom practices, they release the incessant distortions of everyday thinking to lead enlightened lives. The seven wisdom traditions are:

- Practice a consciousness discipline, such as meditation.
- Reduce cravings and find the soul's desire.
- Cultivate emotional wisdom: heal emotional wounds and learn to love.
- Live ethically.
- Awaken the spiritual vision and see the sacred in all things.
- Cultivate spiritual intelligence: the wisdom to understand life.
- Express spirit in action: embrace generosity and the joy of service.

I hope you'll come to see self-hypnosis as a consciousness discipline in the wisdom tradition. I believe that such disciplines can bring about an ongoing transformation of identity. In addition to meditation and self-hypnosis, consciousness disciplines might include body awareness practices such as yoga and dance, participating in music and the visual arts, prayer, reading inspirational literature, journaling, contemplating nature, and spending time with animals. Such practices contribute to personal mastery because they allow us rest, recover from daily pressures, and renew our energies. We need relaxation and down-time.

In *The Power of Full Engagement*, Jim Loehr and Tony Schwartz wrote that the world we live in sometimes seems hostile to rest and renewal: "a world that celebrates work and activity, ignores renewal and recovery, and fails to recognize that both are necessary for sustained high performance."[92] Advances in technology, meant to help us stay connected with one another, often serve to keep us from disconnecting – from each other and from machines and appliances. The information overload and the constant sense of being available sap our attention and energies, overriding our natural, biological rhythms.

Loehr and Schwartz suggested that our capacity to be fully engaged depends on our ability to periodically disengage. We must learn to build stopping points into each day for contemplation, introspection, and psychological recovery from stress. Without such practices, we develop symptoms, negative emotions, and unwanted habits. Practices reveal the connection of the body, mind, and spirit. They provide us with insight, awareness, energy, and inspiration for our callings. Practices sharpen us for the "inner game" of life. I hope self-hypnosis becomes one your practices.

Endnotes

Chapter 1 – Hypnosis: Where Did It Come From?

1. Hull, C. 2002. *Hypnosis and Suggestibility: An Experimental Approach* (reprint edn). Bancyfelin, Wales: Crown House Publishing.
2. Elman, D. 1964. *Hypnotherapy*. Glendale, CA: Westwood Publishing Company.

Chapter 2 – What is Hypnosis Exactly?

3. Jamieson G. A. (ed.) 2007. *Hypnosis and Conscious States: The Cognitive Neuroscience Perspective*. Oxford: Oxford University Press.
4. Gurgevich, S. 2005. *Self-Hypnosis Home Study Course*. Boulder, CO: Sounds True, Inc.
5. Rawlings, R. M. 1997. The genetics of hypnotizability. Unpublished doctoral dissertation, University of New South Wales.
6. Bonnington, S., Tang, B. K., Hawkin, M. B., and Gruzelier, J. H. 2006. Relaxation strategies and enhancement of hypnotic susceptibility. *Brain Research Bulletin* 11;71 (1–3): 83–90.

Chapter 3 – An Overview of NLP

7. NLP trainers L. Michael Hall and Bob Bodenhamer refer to these qualities of internal experience as "meta-details," based on Bandler and Grinder's observation that people must go "meta" to internal experiences in order to examine them. See Hall, L. M. and Bodenhamer, B. G. 1999. *The Structure of Excellence*. Grand Junction, CO: Society for Neuro-Semantics.
8. Bodenhamer B. G. and Hall, L. M. 1997. *Time Lining: Patterns for Adventuring in Time*. Bancyfelin, Wales: Anglo-American Book Company.

Chapter 4 – Mind Magic: Affirmation and Visualization

9. Brooks, C. H. 1923. *The Practice of Autosuggestion by the Method of Émile Coué*. London: George Allen and Unwin.
10. Fisher, H. 2002. *The Fifteen-Minute Miracle*. Austin, TX: Affrm Productions.
11. Andreas, S. 2008. *Help With Negative Self-talk, Vol 1*, Chapter 4, "Talking to Yourself Positively." (e-book) http://www.realpeoplepress.com/pages.php?page=selftalkebook.
12. Simonton, S. M., Simonton, O. C., and Creighton, J. L. 1978. *Getting Well Again*. New York: J. P. Tarcher.
13. Epstein, G. 1989. *Healing Visualization: Creating Health through Imagery*. New York: Bantam Books.

14. Pascual-Leone, A., Nguyet, D., Cohen, L. G., Brasil-Neto, J. P., Cammarota, A., and Hallett, M. 1995. Modulation of muscle responses evoked by transcranial magnetic stimulation during the acquisition of new motor skills. *Journal of Neurophysiology* 74(3): 1037–1045.

15. Murphy, S. 1990. Models of imagery in sport psychology: a review. *Journal of Mental Imagery* 14(3–4): 153–172.

16. Fisher, H. *The Fifteen-Minute Miracle*. Austin, TX: Affrm Productions.

Chapter 5 – Inducing and Deepening Trance

17. Rossi, E. L. and Lippincott, B. 1993. A clinical-experimental exploration of Erickson's naturalistic approach: ultradian time and trance phenomena. *Hypnos* 20: 10–20.

18. Gurgevich, S. 2005. *Self-Hypnosis Home Study Course*. Boulder, CO: Sounds True, Inc.

19. While there are many variations on this induction, I learned the Staircase Induction from James Ramey of Ultra Depth® International.

Part II – Practical Applications in Self-Hypnosis

20. This self-image pattern was inspired by the NLP Swish Pattern, found in Bandler, R. 1985. *Using Your Brain for a Change*. Moab, UT: Real People Press.

Chapter 6 – Eliminate Unwanted Habits and Addictions

21. Covey, S. 1994. *First Things First*. New York: Simon & Schuster.

22. Doidge, N. 2007. *The Brain that Changes Itself*. New York: Penguin.

23. Prochaska, J. O. 1979. *Systems of Psychotherapy: A Transtheoretical Analysis*. Homewood, IL: Dorsey Press.

24. Bandler, R. and Grinder, J. 1982. *Reframing: Neuro-Linguistic Programming and the Transformation of Meaning*. Moab, UT: Real People Press.

25. Hall, L. M. 2000. *Secrets of Personal Mastery*. Bancyfelin, Wales: Crown House Publishing.

26. Morewedge, C. K., Huh, Y. E., and Vosgerau, J. 2010. Thought for food: imagined consumption reduces actual consumption. *Science* 333 (6010): 1530–1533.

Chapter 7 – Yes, You *Can* Stop Smoking!

27. Since 1988, I've studied and taught NLP with Ron Klein, Certified NLP trainer and Director of the American Hypnosis Training Academy, in Silver Spring, Maryland.

28. This step is recommended in Botsford, D. 2007. *Hypnosis for Smoking Cessation: An NLP and Hypnotherapy Practitioner's Manual*. Bancyfelin, Wales: Crown House Publishing.

Chapter 8 – Achieve Your Ideal Weight

29. Taubes, G. 2008. The diet that really works, and why most others don't. *Bottom Line Personal*, February, pp. 13–14.
30. Appleton, N. 2010. Suicide by sugar. *Bottom Line Secrets*, July, pp. 3–5.
31. Many of these recommendations are drawn from Corsetty, K. and Pearson, J. 2000. *Healthy Habits: Total Conditioning for a Healthy Body and Mind*. Lincoln, NE: Dageforde Publishing.
32. Andreas, C. and Andreas, S. 1989. *Heart of the Mind*. Moab, UT: Real People Press.

Chapter 9 – Quality Sleep

33. Breus, M. 2011. *The Sleep Doctor's Diet Plan: Lose Weight Through Better Sleep*. New York: Rodale, Inc.
34. In *Los Angeles Times*, Saturday, April 4, 2009. Sleeping pill use grows as economy keeps people up at night. The source of the statistic was IMS Health, a health research corporation.
35. Sources:
    - Harvey, J. R. 2001. *Deep Sleep*. New York: M. Evans and Company, Inc.
    - National Center for Sleep Disorders, April 2006. *Your Guide to Healthy Sleep*. U.S. Department of Health and Human Services, National Institutes of Health.
    - Worwood, V. A. 1991. *The Complete Book of Essential Oils and Aromatherapy*. Novato, CA: New World Library.

Chapter 10 – Start Exercising!

36. Much of this chapter is drawn from Corsetty, K. and Pearson, J. 2000. *Healthy Habits: Total Conditioning for a Healthy Body and Mind*. Lincoln, NE: Dageforde Publishing.
37. Van Praag, H., Shubert, T., Zhao, C., and Gage, F. H. 2005. Exercise enhances learning and hippocampal neurogenesis in aged mice. *Journal of Neuroscience* 25(38): 8680–8685.
38. Sources:
    - Cameron-Bandler, L., Gordon, D., and Lebeau, M. 1985. *Know How: Guided Programs for Inventing Your Own Best Future*. San Rafael, CA: FuturePace, Inc.
    - O'Connor, J. and Seymour, J. 1990. *Introducing Neuro-Linguistic Programming*. London: Mandala.
    - Hall, L. M. and Belnap, B. R. 2004. *The Sourcebook of Magic: A Comprehensive Guide to NLP Change Patterns* (2nd edn). Bancyfelin, Wales: Crown House Publishing.
    - Grinder, J. and Bandler, R. 1981. *Trance-Formations: Neuro-Linguistic Programming and the Structure of Hypnosis*. Moab, UT: Real People Press.

Chapter 11 – Maximize Your Motivation!

39. Covey, S. 1989. *The Seven Habits of Highly Effective People*. New York: Simon & Schuster.

40. Maurer, R. 2004. *One Small Step Can Change Your Life: The Kaizen Way*. New York: Workman Publishing.

41. See Miller, J. 2004. *The Question Behind the Question*. New York: Putnam; and Miller, J. 2006. *Flipping the Switch*. New York: Putnam.

42. Ellis, D. 2002. *Falling Awake: Creating the Life of Your Dreams*. Rapid City, SD: Breakthrough Enterprises.

43. McDermott, I. and Jago, W. 2001. *The NLP Coach*. London: Piatkus.

44. de Shazer, S. 1988. *Clues: Investigating Solutions in Brief Therapy*. New York: W. W. Norton.

45. This strategy was adapted from Overdurf, J. and Silverthorn, J. 1995. *Training Trances: Multi-Level Communication in Therapy and Training* (3rd edn). Portland, OR: Metamorphous Press; and Grinder, J. and Bandler, R. 1981. *Trance-Formations: Neuro-Linguistic Programming and the Structure of Hypnosis*. Moab, UT: Real People Press.

Chapter 12 – Stop Procrastinating Once and For All!

46. Covey, S. 1994. *First Things First*. New York: Simon & Schuster.

47. Lakein, A. 1989. *How to Get Control of Your Time and Your Life*. New York: Signet.

48. In Hall, L. M. and Belnap, B. R. 2004. *The Sourcebook of Magic: A Comprehensive Guide to NLP Change Patterns* (2nd edn). Bancyfelin, Wales: Crown House Publishing.

49. Hall, L. M. 2000. *Secrets of Personal Mastery*. Bancyfelin, Wales: Crown House Publishing.

50. Pearson, P. 1998. *Stop Self-Sabotage! How to Get Out of Your Own Way and Have an Extraordinary Life*. Newport Coast, CA: Connemara Press.

Chapter 13 – Improve Your Performance

51. Edgette, J. H. and Rowan, T. 2003. *Winning the Mind Game: Using Hypnosis in Sport Psychology*. Bancyfelin, Wales: Crown House Publishing.

52. Adapted from Andreas, C. and Andreas, S. 1989. *Heart of the Mind*. Moab, UT: Real People Press.

Chapter 14 – Pass Your Polygraph Exam

No endnotes for this chapter.

Chapter 15 – Give Your Self-Esteem a Lift!

53. Hansen, B. 2006. *Shame and Anger: The Criticism Connection*. Washington, DC: Change for Good Press.

54. Goldsmith, C. 2003. *The Book of Carols*. Haverford, PA: Infinity Publishing.

55. Hay, L. L. 1984. *You Can Heal Your Life*. Santa Monica, CA: Hay House.

56. Hall, L. M. 2000. *Accessing Personal Genius Training Manual*. Grand Junction, CO: Neuro-Semantics Publications.

57. McDonald, R. 1979. *The Walking Belief Change Pattern* (audio cassette). Boulder, CO: NLP Comprehensive.

58. In Hall, L. M. and Belnap, B. R. 2004. *The Sourcebook of Magic: A Comprehensive Guide to NLP Change Patterns* (2nd edn). Bancyfelin, Wales: Crown House Publishing.

Chapter 16 – Manage Your Emotions for Equanimity and Resilience

59. Most of these recommendations originally came from Corsetty, K. and Pearson, J. 2000. *Healthy Habits: Total Conditioning for a Healthy Body and Mind*. Lincoln, NE: Dageforde Publishing.

60. Walsh, P. 2007. *It's All Too Much: An Easy Plan for Living a Better Life with Less Stuff*. New York: Free Press.

61. Kemp, N. 2008. In Steve Andreas's NLP email newsletter (no title).

62. In Bodenhamer, B. 2004. *Mastering Blocking and Stuttering: A Cognitive Approach to Achieving Fluency*. Bancyfelin, Wales: Crown House Publishing.

63. This NLP pattern goes by additional names, such as Visual Squash, Parts Negotiation, and Parts Integration. Sources:
    - Classroom notes from Klein, R. 2005. *Level II Ericksonian Hypnosis and Brief Therapy Training*. Silver Spring, MD: American Hypnosis Training Academy.
    - Andreas, C. and Andreas S. 1989. *Heart of the Mind*. Moab, UT: Real People Press.
    - O'Connor, J. and Seymour, J. 1990. *Introducing Neuro-Linguistic Programming*. London: Mandala.

Chapter 17 – Pain Management and Relief

64. Crawford, H. J. 1994. Brain dynamics and hypnosis: attentional and disattentional abilities. *International Journal of Clinical and Experimental Hypnosis* 42: 204–232.

65. Pert, C. B. 2006. *Everything You Need To Know To Feel Go(o)d*. Carlsbad, CA: Hay House.

66. Spiegel, D. and Bloom, J. R. 1983. Group therapy and hypnosis reduce metastatic breast carcinoma pain. *Psychosomatic Medicine* 45(4): 333–339; and Syrjala, K. L., Cummings, C., and Donaldson, G. W. 1992. Hypnosis or cognitive behavioral training for the reduction of pain and nausea during cancer treatment: a controlled clinical trial. *Pain* 48: 137–146.

67. Patterson, D. R., Everett, J. J., Burns, G. L., and Marvin, J. A. 1992. Hypnosis for the treatment of burn pain. *Journal of Consulting and Clinical Psychology* 60: 713–717.

68. Hannen, H. C. M., Hoenderdos, H. T. W., Van Romunde, L. K. J., Hop, W. C. J., Malle, C., Terwiel, J. P., and Hekster, G. B. 1991. Controlled trial of hypnotherapy in the treatment of refractory fibromyalgia. *Journal of Rheumatology* 18(1): 72–75.

69. Patterson, D. R. and Jensen, M. P. 2003. Hypnosis and clinical pain. *Psychology Bulletin* 129(4): 495–521.

70. Eimer, B. N. 2008. *Hypnotize Yourself Out Of Pain Now!* (2nd edn). Bancyfelin, Wales: Crown House Publishing.

71. Brigham, D. D. 1996. *Imagery for Getting Well: Clinical Applications of Behavioral Medicine*. New York: W. W. Norton.

Chapter 18 – Preparing for Surgery or Medical Procedures

72. Ginandes, C. S., Brooks, P., Sando, W., Jones, C., and Aker, J. 2002. Can medical hypnosis accelerate post-surgical wound healing? Results of a clinical trial. *American Journal of Clinical Hypnosis* 45(4): 333–351; and Ginandes, C. S. and Rosenthal, D. I. 1999. Using hypnosis to accelerate the healing of bone fractures. *Alternative Therapies in Health and Medicine* 5(2): 67–75.

73. Montgomery, G. H., Bovbjerg, D. H., Schnur, J. B., David, D., Goldfarb, A., Weltz, C. R., Schechter. C., Graff-Zivin, J., Tatrow, K., Price, D. D., and Silverstein, J. H. 2007. A randomized clinical trial of a brief hypnosis intervention to control side effects in breast surgery patients. *Journal of the National Cancer Institute* 99(17): 1304–1312.

74. Lang, E. V., Benotsch, E. G., Fick, L. J., Lutgendorf, S., Berbaum, M. L., Berbaum, K., S, Logan, H., and Spiegel, D. 2000. Adjunct non-pharmacologic analgesia for invasive medical procedures: A randomized trial. *The Lancet* 355: 1486–1490.

75. Siegel, B. S. 1988. *Love, Medicine and Miracles* (audio cassette). New York: Caedmon.

76. This originally appeared in Pearson, J. 1996. Helping Clients Prepare for Medical Procedures. *Anchor Point*, Vol. 10 (11) pp. 14–23.

Chapter 19 – Heal Emotional Hurts Connected with the Past

77. James, T. and Woodsmall, W. 1988. *Time Line Therapy and the Basis of Personality*. Cupertino, CA: Meta Publications.

78. Bodenhamer, B. G. and Hall, L. M. 1997. *Time Lining: Patterns for Adventuring in Time*. Bancyfelin, Wales: Anglo-American Book Company.

79. Bandler, R. and Grinder, J. 1979. *Frogs into Princes*. Moab, UT: Real People Press.

80. Andreas, C. 1992. *Advanced Language Patterns* (audio cassette). Boulder, CO: NLP Comprehensive.

81. Andreas, C. and Andreas, S. 1991. A Brief History of NLP. *The Vak*, Volume X, No 1, Winter 1991–92, p. 1.

82. Dilts, R. 1990. *Changing Belief Systems with NLP*. Cupertino, CA: Meta Publications.

Chapter 20 – Access Your Intuitive Wisdom

83. Moss, R. 1996. *Conscious Dreaming: A Spiritual Path for Everyday Life*. New York: Crown Trade Paperbacks.

84. O'Hanlon-Hudson, P. 1993. *Making Friends with Your Unconscious Mind*. Omaha, NE: Center Press.

85. Kinser, P. 2007. *Limitless Living: An Unconventional Guide to Spiritual Exploration and Growth*. Montross, VA: Ancient Otter Publishing.

Chapter 21 – Define Your Life Purpose

86. Allen, J. 1903. *As a Man Thinketh*. This book is in the public domain and has been reproduced in book form and on websites.

87. O'Hanlon, W. 2009. *Let Your Soul Be Your Pilot: Finding Your Direction in Life* (audio CD). Bancyfelin, Wales: Crown House Publishing.

88. Gilligan, S. and Dilts, R. 2009. *The Hero's Journey*. Bancyfelin, Wales: Crown House Publishing.

89. Hass, R.A. 2003. Using perceptual positions to ask "What is your soul dream?" *Anchor Point*, April, pp. 34–37. Many thanks to the author for her comments on my adaptation.

90. Frankl, V. E. 1963. *Man's Search for Meaning: An Introduction to Logotherapy*, tr. I. Lasch. New York: Washington Square Press.

Afterword

91. Walsh, R. 1999. *Essential Spirituality: The 7 Central Practices to Awaken Heart and Mind*. New York: John Wiley.

92. Loehr, J. and Schwartz, T. 2003. *The Power of Full Engagement*. New York: Free Press.

References

Andreas, C. 1992. *Advanced Language Patterns* (audio cassette). Boulder, CO: NLP Comprehensive.

Andreas, S. 2008. *Help With Negative Self-talk, Vol 1*, Chapter 4, "Talking to Yourself Positively." (e-book) http://www.realpeoplepress.com/pages.php?page=selftalkebook.

Andreas, C. and Andreas, S. 1989. *Heart of the Mind*. Moab, UT: Real People Press.

Andreas, C. and Andreas, S. 1991. A Brief History of NLP. *The Vak*, Volume X, No 1, Winter 1991–92, p. 1.

Appleton, N. 2010. Suicide by sugar. *Bottom Line Secrets*, July, pp. 3–5.

Bandler, R. 1985. *Using Your Brain for a Change*. Moab, UT: Real People Press.

Bandler, R. and Grinder, J. 1979. *Frogs into Princes*. Moab, UT: Real People Press.

Bandler, R. and Grinder, J. 1982. *Reframing: Neuro-Linguistic Programming and the Transformation of Meaning*. Moab, UT: Real People Press.

Bodenhamer, B. 2004. *Mastering Blocking and Stuttering: A Cognitive Approach to Achieving Fluency*. Bancyfelin, Wales: Crown House Publishing.

Bodenhamer B. G. and Hall, L. M. 1997. *Time Lining: Patterns for Adventuring in Time*. Bancyfelin, Wales: Anglo-American Book Company.

Bonnington, S., Tang, B. K., Hawkin, M. B., and Gruzelier, J. H. 2006. Relaxation strategies and enhancement of hypnotic susceptibility. *Brain Research Bulletin* 11;71(1–3): 83–90.

Botsford, D. 2007. *Hypnosis for Smoking Cessation: An NLP and Hypnotherapy Practitioner's Manual*. Bancyfelin, Wales: Crown House Publishing.

Breus, M. 2011. *The Sleep Doctor's Diet Plan: Lose Weight Through Better Sleep*. New York: Rodale, Inc.

Brigham, D. D. 1996. *Imagery for Getting Well: Clinical Applications of Behavioral Medicine*. New York: W. W. Norton.

Brooks, C. H. 1923. *The Practice of Autosuggestion by the Method of Émile Coué*. London: George Allen and Unwin.

Cameron-Bandler, L., Gordon, D., and Lebeau, M. 1985. *Know How: Guided Programs for Inventing Your Own Best Future*. San Rafael, CA: FuturePace, Inc.

Corsetty, K. and Pearson, J. 2000. *Healthy Habits: Total Conditioning for a Healthy Body and Mind*. Lincoln, NE: Dageforde Publishing.

Covey, S. 1989. *The Seven Habits of Highly Effective People*. New York: Simon & Schuster.

Covey, S. 1994. *First Things First*. New York: Simon & Schuster.

Crawford, H. J. 1994. Brain dynamics and hypnosis: attentional and disattentional abilities. *International Journal of Clinical and Experimental Hypnosis* 42: 204–232.

de Shazer, S. 1988. *Clues: Investigating Solutions in Brief Therapy*. New York: W. W. Norton.

Dilts, R. 1990. *Changing Belief Systems with NLP*. Cupertino, CA: Meta Publications.

Doidge, N. 2007. *The Brain that Changes Itself*. New York: Penguin.

Edgette, J. H. and Rowan, T. 2003. *Winning the Mind Game: Using Hypnosis in Sport Psychology*. Bancyfelin, Wales: Crown House Publishing.

Eimer, B. N. 2008. *Hypnotize Yourself Out of Pain Now!* (2nd edn). Bancyfelin, Wales: Crown House Publishing.

Ellis, D. 2002. *Falling Awake: Creating the Life of Your Dreams*. Rapid City, SD: Breakthrough Enterprises.

Elman, D. 1964. *Hypnotherapy*. Glendale, CA: Westwood Publishing Company.

Epstein, G. 1989. *Healing Visualization: Creating Health through Imagery*. New York: Bantam Books.

Fisher, H. 2002. *The Fifteen-Minute Miracle*. Austin, TX: Affrm Productions.

Frankl, V. E. 1963. *Man's Search for Meaning: An Introduction to Logotherapy*, tr. I. Lasch. New York: Washington Square Press.

Gellene, D. April 4, 2009. Sleeping pill use grows as economy keeps people up at night. *Los Angeles Times*. http://www.latimes.com/features/health/la-he-sleep30-2009mar30,0,1418832.story

Gilligan, S. and Dilts, R. 2009. *The Hero's Journey*. Bancyfelin, Wales: Crown House Publishing.

Ginandes C. S., Brooks, P., Sando, W., Jones, C., and Aker, J. 2002. Can medical hypnosis accelerate post-surgical wound healing? Results of a clinical trial. *American Journal of Clinical Hypnosis* 45(4): 333–351.

Ginandes, C. S. and Rosenthal, D. I. 1999. Using hypnosis to accelerate the healing of bone fractures. *Alternative Therapies in Health and Medicine* 5(2): 67–75.

Goldsmith, C. 2003. *The Book of Carols*. Haverford, PA: Infinity Publishing.

Grinder, J. and Bandler, R. 1981. *Trance-Formations: Neuro-Linguistic Programming and the Structure of Hypnosis*. Moab, UT: Real People Press.

Gurgevich, S. 2005. *Self-Hypnosis Home Study Course*. Boulder, CO: Sounds True, Inc.

Hall, L. M. 2000. *Accessing Personal Genius Training Manual*. Grand Junction, CO: Neuro-Semantics Publications.

Hall, L. M. 2000. *Secrets of Personal Mastery*. Bancyfelin, Wales: Crown House Publishing.

Hall, L. M. and Belnap, B. R. 2004. *The Sourcebook of Magic: A Comprehensive Guide to NLP Change Patterns* (2nd edn). Bancyfelin, Wales: Crown House Publishing.

Hall, L. M. and Bodenhamer, B. G. 1999. *The Structure of Excellence*. Grand Junction, CO: Society for Neuro-Semantics

Hannen, H. C. M., Hoenderdos, H. T. W., Van Romunde, L. K. J., Hop, W. C. J., Malle, C., Terwiel, J. P., and Hekster, G. B. 1991. Controlled trial of hypnotherapy in the treatment of refractory fibromyalgia. *Journal of Rheumatology* 18(1): 72–75.

Hansen, B. 2006. *Shame and Anger: The Criticism Connection*. Washington, DC: Change for Good Press.

Harvey, J. R. 2001. *Deep Sleep*. New York: M. Evans and Company, Inc.

Hass, R. A. 2003. Using perceptual positions to ask "What is your soul dream?" *Anchor Point*, April, pp. 34–37.

Hay, L. L. 1984. *You Can Heal Your Life*. Santa Monica, CA: Hay House.

Hull, C. 2002. *Hypnosis and Suggestibility: An Experimental Approach* (reprint edn). Bancyfelin, Wales: Crown House Publishing.

James, T. and Woodsmall, W. 1988. *Time Line Therapy and the Basis of Personality*. Cupertino, CA: Meta Publications.

Jamieson G. A. (ed.) 2007. *Hypnosis and Conscious States: The Cognitive Neuroscience Perspective*. Oxford: Oxford University Press.

Kinser, P. 2007. *Limitless Living: An Unconventional Guide to Spiritual Exploration and Growth*. Montross, VA: Ancient Otter Publishing.

Lakein, A. 1989. *How to Get Control of Your Time and Your Life*. New York: Signet.

Lang, E. V., Benotsch, E. G., Fick, L. J., Lutgendorf, S., Berbaum, M. L., Berman, K. S., Logan, H., and Spiegel, D. 2000. Adjunct non-pharmacologic analgesia for invasive medical procedures: a randomized trial. *The Lancet* 355: 1486–1490.

Loehr, J. and Schwartz, T. 2003. *The Power of Full Engagement*. New York: Free Press.

McDermott, I. and Jago, W. 2001. *The NLP Coach*. London: Piatkus.

McDonald, R. 1979. *The Walking Belief Change Pattern* (audio cassette). Boulder, CO: NLP Comprehensive.

Maurer, R. 2004, *One Small Step Can Change Your Life: The Kaizen Way*. New York: Workman Publishing.

Miller, J. 2004. *The Question behind the Question*. New York: Putnam.

Miller, J. 2006. *Flipping the Switch*. New York: Putnam.

Montgomery, G. H., Bovbjerg, D. H., Schnur, J. B., David, D., Goldfarb, A., Weltz, C. R., Schechter. C., Graff-Zivin, J., Tatrow, K., Price, D. D., and Silverstein, J. H. 2007. A randomized clinical trial of a brief hypnosis intervention to control side effects in breast surgery patients. *Journal of the National Cancer Institute* 99(17): 1304–1312.

Morewedge, C. K., Huh, Y. E., and Vosgerau, J. 2010. Thought for food: imagined consumption reduces actual consumption. *Science* 333(6010): 1530–1533.

Moss, R. 1996. *Conscious Dreaming: A Spiritual Path for Everyday Life*. New York: Crown Trade Paperbacks.

Murphy, S. 1990. Models of imagery in sport psychology: a review. *Journal of Mental Imagery* 14(3–4): 153–172.

National Center for Sleep Disorders. 2006. *Your Guide to Healthy Sleep* (pdf). U.S. Department of Health and Human Services, National Institutes of Health.

O'Connor, J. and Seymour, J. 1990. *Introducing Neuro-Linguistic Programming*. London: Mandala.

O'Hanlon, W. 2009. *Let Your Soul Be Your Pilot: Finding Your Direction in Life* (audio CD). Bancyfelin, Wales: Crown House Publishing.

O'Hanlon-Hudson, P. 1993. *Making Friends with Your Unconscious Mind*. Omaha, NE: Center Press.

Overdurf, J. and Silverthorn, J. 1995. *Training Trances: Multi-Level Communication in Therapy and Training* (3rd edn). Portland, OR: Metamorphous Press.

Pascual-Leone, A., Nguyet, D., Cohen, L. G., Brasil-Neto, J. P., Cammarota, A., and Hallett, M. 1995. Modulation of muscle responses evoked by transcranial magnetic stimulation during the acquisition of new motor skills. *Journal of Neurophysiology* 74(3): 1037–1045.

Patterson, D. R., Everett, J. J., Burns, G. L., and Marvin, J. A. 1992. Hypnosis for the treatment of burn pain. *Journal of Consulting and Clinical Psychology* 60: 713–717.

Patterson, D. R. and Jensen, M. P. 2003. Hypnosis and clinical pain. *Psychology Bulletin* 129(4): 495–521.

Pearson, P. 1998. *Stop Self-Sabotage! How to Get Out of Your Own Way and Have an Extraordinary Life*. Newport Coast, CA: Connemara Press

Pert, C. B. 2006. *Everything You Need to Know to Feel Go(o)d*. Carlsbad, CA: Hay House, Inc.

Prochaska, J. O. 1979. *Systems of Psychotherapy: A Transtheoretical Analysis*. Homewood, IL: Dorsey Press.

Rawlings, R. M. 1997. The genetics of hypnotizability. Unpublished doctoral dissertation, University of New South Wales.

Rossi, E. L. and Lippincott, B. 1993. A clinical-experimental exploration of Erickson's naturalistic approach: ultradian time and trance phenomena. *Hypnos* 20: 10–20.

Siegel, B. S. 1988. *Love, Medicine and Miracles* (audio cassette). New York: Caedmon.

Simonton, S. M., Simonton, O. C., and Creighton, J. L. 1978. *Getting Well Again*. New York: J. P. Tarcher.

Spiegel, D. and Bloom, J. R. 1983. Group therapy and hypnosis reduce metastatic breast carcinoma pain. *Psychosomatic Medicine* 45(4): 333–339.

Syrjala, K. L., Cummings, C., and Donaldson, G. W. 1992. Hypnosis or cognitive behavioral training for the reduction of pain and nausea during cancer treatment: a controlled clinical trial. *Pain* 48: 137–146.

Taubes, G. 2008. The diet that really works, and why most others don't. *Bottom Line Personal*, February, pp. 13–14.

Van Praag, H., Shubert, T., Zhao, C., and Gage, F. H. 2005. Exercise enhances learning and hippocampal neurogenesis in aged mice. *Journal of Neuroscience* 25(38): 8680–8685.

Walsh, P. 2007. *It's All Too Much: An Easy Plan for Living a Better Life with Less Stuff*. New York: Free Press.

Walsh, R. 1999. *Essential Spirituality: The 7 Central Practices to Awaken Heart and Mind*. New York: John Wiley.

Worwood, V. A. 1991. *The Complete Book of Essential Oils and Aromatherapy*. Novato, CA: New World Library.

Index